ARKANA

THIRD LINE MEDICINE

Melvyn Werbach brings to this study his extensive personal experience in both orthodox and alternative medicine. A graduate of Tufts University School of Medicine, Boston, he is a Diplomate of the American Board of Psychiatry and Neurology and a member of the clinical faculty in the Departments of Anesthesiology and Psychiatry at the UCLA School of Medicine, Los Angeles. He is a recipient of the Certificate of Honor of the Biofeedback Society of California 'for making contributions . . . which have altered the development of biofeedback in a positive fashion' and is listed in *Who's Who in the Biobehavioral Sciences* and *Who's Who in the West (USA)*. Doctor Werbach is currently Director of the Biofeedback Medical Clinic in Tarzana, California.

THIRD LINE MEDICINE

MODERN TREATMENT FOR PERSISTENT SYMPTOMS

MELVYN R. WERBACH M.D.

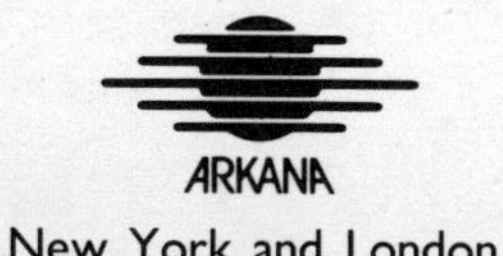

New York and London

First published in 1986
by Arkana Paperbacks
Arkana Paperbacks is an imprint of
Routledge & Kegan Paul Inc.
Published in the USA BY
Routledge & Kegan Paul Inc.
in association with Methuen Inc.
29 West 35th Street, New York, NY 10001

Published in the UK by
Routledge & Kegan Paul plc
11 New Fetter Lane, London EC4P 4EE

Set in 10/11pt. Sabon
by Columns of Reading
and printed in Great Britain
by The Guernsey Press Co. Ltd
Guernsey, Channel Islands

Library of Congress Cataloging in Publication Data
Werbach, Melvyn R.
Third line medicine.

Bibliography: p.
Includes index.
1. Holistic medicine. I. Title.
R733.W46 1986 615.5 85-23277

British Library CIP data also available

ISBN 1-85063-041-0

To my wife, Gail,
and my sons, Kevin and Adam, who have
provided the love and support which made this book possible.

Contents

Foreword

Many, probably most, physicians live by a creed of commitment to the welfare of their patients. There is, as well, a small subgroup whose members believe their perspectives and experience are more suited to teaching and research. These medical professionals are, in effect, indirect healers; they join academic communities to teach and do research. Their therapeutic productivity and confidence lie in the community and its consensus.

There is, fortunately, still another breed of healer. Here and there especially concerned, or sensitive, or intuitive physicians awaken to special circumstances of their patients. They become challenged by incongruous symptoms, by modestly strange and unidentifiable ailments, by uncommon medical events. One patient may show strangely unfamiliar although not life-threatening distress while another may not respond to medically acceptable treatment. These are the healing barriers, and they trouble concerned physicians who find themselves in a therapeutic limbo, backed up against medical points of no-return where sympathy and compassion are the surest aids the healer can provide.

This third kind of healer is the Third Line Physician. This is the healer whose commitment cannot accept healing barriers and whose mind meets these medical challenges with a nip and a tweak of every reservoir of professional therapeutic acumen.

Pursuing diagnoses and treatment possibilities when all else has failed requires not merely persistence and devotion, but it requires, as well, an exquisite sensitivity to the patient's world and being. The reward for this dedicated pursuit of therapeutic promise is the relief of a patient's illness.

Happily, in the past decade or so new (and renewed) perceptions of the nature of human ills and states of wellness have been evolving. As with anything else undergoing evolution, some evolving insights can be useful while many are not. At first, for example, medical orthodoxy accepted dietary deficiencies or allergies only when very narrowly defined, while such foreign procedures as acupuncture or yoga or autogenic training were looked upon as practices to be eschewed. Much has now been sorted out and the bulk of medical opinion has come to recognize that the world has indeed changed and that human beings are more psychobiologically complex and more immunologically different than ever before believed. Only in the past decade has modern man become convinced that mind and body interact, that mind and body grow together and work together and can heal and care for each other. It was the Novelist Roger Sperry who wrote nearly fifteen years ago that life-long neuropsychological studies led him to conclude that just as brain events affect mental events, so do mental events affect the neural activities of the brain. There is more to health and illness than just physical elements.*

In *Third Line Medicine* Dr. Werbach describes the profound effect of medical traditions on health and illness. Years ago malfunction caused body changes we could identify as illness. Then, by a process of deduction, we could identify the cause or the treatment or both.

But times have changed – radically. Nearly everything in the world can come into contact with virtually everything else in the universe. Viruses, unseen toxins, virulent social values or even radical environments can whistle by and we ourselves move through them, unaware of their hidden dangers. Travellers and the pathologies they host move into and through new environments of countries and space, while communications, loaded with persuasions and lures move with the speed of light. Exposure is a new phenomenon of life that puts modern man dead center in the arena of a new and immensely broad assortment of hurts and ills and psychic assaults. Today we are exposed totally – mind and body, eyes and ears, nose and skin, feelings and memories and immune life support systems – all are exposed more today than ever before. It is understandable that we face new and different, more complex and subtle and

*Sperry, R.W. An objective approach to subjective experiences: further explanation of a hypothesis. *Psychol. Rev.* 77:585-90,1970

more resistant ailments and distress.

It is a time for Third Line Medicine. It is, however, a difficult phenomenon to write about. There is no doubt that our understanding of the nature of health is changing rapidly across the many dimensions that we are learning to determine illness and wellness. Still, it is difficult to write about a tradition when its perceptions seem to be changing markedly and especially when so many of its healing practices are cloaked in conservatism. As Dr. Werbach very capably describes, the history of medicine is a history of how the feelings of health and illness became replaced by objective physical or chemical or immunological signs, and how medicine lost sight of the notion of the integrity and wholeness and harmony of being that Hippocrates himself saw as the foundations of health. All medicine grew from study of the pathological (from serious illness), not from study of the dynamics of wellness. Even psychotherapy and psychiatry are built up from a base of pathology, not from consideration of the integrated being or a psychological immune system and the role it plays in health and wellness.

Medicine has seen more change these past two decades than at any time during its entire history. Recent medical research has produced more than its share of benefits, yet the practice of medicine continues to suffer severely from a succession of distracting socio-economic factors. The pressures of such non-therapeutic intrusions as cost-effective considerations of drugs or hospital care, malpractice insurance, over-specialization, even 'morality' ailments have all worked to undermine the universal perception of healing as a dynamic interrelationship between healer and the unwell.

Rethinking medicine is a modern imperative, and while nearly everyone recognizes the need, few can respond. It is a long and arduous task to analyze one of the most powerful traditions of all history, to describe its flaws objectively, then try to begin to lay the foundations for mending its imperfections. It takes a good bit of courage to self-examine one's professional base and a good bit more patience and determination to define the good and the bad and work out ways to reconstruct theoretical foundations and the building blocks that can lead to improving the arts and sciences of healing.

You will note that Dr. Werbach critiques primarily the

scientific fallacies of traditional medicine and the rigidity and narrowness they foster and he uses the precise data and argument of science itself. He not only documents some of the most far-reaching errors of popular medical practice, he dissects them. He also describes a host of rarely investigated causative factors of illness and unwellness, such as allergies more obscure than hay fever, hidden toxicities, unrecognized sensitivities to different kinds of elements and other causes of illness that fall between the cracks of traditional medicine. He provides some fascinating case reports that illustrate the medical sleuthing the physician needs to do in order to practice Third Line Medicine and he gives us new insights into the 'nondisease' suffering so many must endure because of the rigid conventions and limitations of outdated medical doctrine that too often sees its use as a medical security blanket.

This book probes why many traditions of medical practice need to be examined. Moreover, it suggests how to use this new understanding to produce a more humane, more caring and more therapeutically effective professional community, a community of professional healers especially equipped to heal those unwell with needs for a broader and more individually relevant therapeutic base than First or Second Line Medicine can provide.

And, as just one more sign of his concern for victims of illness. Dr. Werbach ends his contribution to modern medicine with an appendix designed to guide the reader toward finding competent third line practitioners.

Barbara B. Brown
Rancho Santa Fe, California

Acknowledgments

There are many ways in which people influence others. While speeches, articles and books have their effects, nothing is as powerful as is the personal influence of friends and colleagues who challenge us to open our eyes to new ideas and support us when our own ideas run counter to prevailing thought. People in my life who have done that for me include John Ackerman, M.D., David E. Bresler, Ph.D. and the entire staff of the former UCLA Pain Control Unit, Barbara B. Brown, Ph.D., Hyla Cass, M.D., Roger Coger, Ph.D., Jackie Diamond, M.S.W., Lewis Mayron, Ph.D., Eugene Roberts, Ph.D. and Jack Sandweiss, M.A..

Each of them, by enthusiastically participating with me in numerous informal discussions of issues raised in this book, has contributed to its contents, and I am grateful.

CHAPTER 1
The third line concept

It is more important to know what sort of
person has a disease than to know what sort
of disease a person has.

HIPPOCRATES
460–377 BC

A physician is obligated to consider
more than a diseased organ, more even
than the whole man – he must view
the man in his world.

HARVEY CUSHING
1869–1939
(Quoted by René Dubos in
Man Adapting, Chapter 12)

It has been five years now since her pain became so intense that Alice sought the help of her family doctor. After he examined and tested her, he gave her medications which relieved some of the pain, but also made her groggy. She soon decided that they were not worth taking and stopped them.

At her next visit, he referred her to a colleague who specialized in the treatment of similar problems. The colleague put her through more tests, tried further treatments which did little to help her, and eventually sent her back to her family physician. Some time passed, and Alice, who was getting worse, was referred to a surgeon who suggested surgery. Feeling desperate, she agreed.

She now regrets her decision. Surgery changed the pain somewhat, but did not make it better. Her family doctor has suggested that she see a psychiatrist, but Alice has refused as she knows that her pain is real, and therefore doesn't believe that talking can make it better. She feels depressed, has become irritable with her family, and has withdrawn from her friends.

Alice is a candidate for Third Line Medicine.

Despite our hope of maintaining robust good health until the day of our demise, most people will experience periods of illness in their lives which are of sufficient concern that they seek medical assistance. Generally, they approach first their family physicians for that assistance. These physicians provide an evaluation of the illness and, if they feel competent to deal with it themselves, render the appropriate treatment. Soon, if all goes well, the illness remits sufficiently so that both physicians and patients agree that no further professional care is indicated.

General practitioners used to provide front line services, but today GPs are a dying species, having been increasingly replaced by more highly trained, and often more specialized, physicians. Their replacements include family practitioners, pediatricians, and internists, all of whom, in addition to any specialty interests, can be said to practice First Line Medicine.

There are times when these physicians conclude that their backgrounds are inadequate for the proper evaluation or treatment of the illness. In these cases, they refer their patients to one or more specialists whose practices are restricted to a more limited aspect of medical diagnosis or treatment. These specialists provide a second line of medical care and operate quite differently from their first line counterparts. While first line physicians attempt to view the illness in a comprehensive manner, second line physicians are sharply focused upon those aspects of the illness which relate to their area of specialization.

Once patients enter the field of Second Line Medicine, they may only see one specialist, or they may end up by seeing several. The illness may now remit due to their interventions and they may return to the care of their first line physicians, or perhaps they will face one disappointment after another as each specialist fails to discover a treatment which produces an acceptable degree of relief at an acceptable personal cost.

Eventually, in the latter case, further consultations with additional specialists become fruitless. The recommendations of the second line physicians have either been followed, but to no avail, or they have been refused. If surgery had seemed to be the answer, all appropriate operations would have been performed. If medications had seemed to be the answer, all appropriate drugs would have been tried. If psychiatric care had seemed to be the answer, it had either been refused or it had not resulted in improvement. If physical therapy had seemed to be the answer, a trial of various physical modalities of treatment would have failed to give adequate relief.

Traditionally, these unfortunate people have had two options. The first was to give up hope of ever feeling better. If they chose this option, they returned to the exclusive care of their front line physicians and took on the task of 'learning to live with' their symptoms. This has been the option usually recommended by their physicians, and thus those who have selected it have complied with their doctors' wishes.

Some of these people have subsequently done relatively well. The conviction that they have done all that they could do to find an effective treatment helps them to refocus their lives away from their symptoms and towards finding gratifications which counterbalance their distress. Others, who are less able to cope, preoccupy themselves with their symptoms and remain chronically depressed.

The second option was to refuse to accept their physicians' resignation in the battle against the illness by continuing to seek relief and possible cure from those who offered it. This has meant going outside the medical profession to enlist the services of a wide assortment of both licensed and unlicensed health care practitioners.

Those who chose this option were faced with a dilemma. While they were being evaluated and treated by the medical profession, their concerns over receiving appropriate treatment were minimized by that profession's broad consensus as to acceptable medical practices. This was true even when they traveled from specialist to specialist, as each physician they consulted usually respected the knowledge of his or her colleagues even when there was a specific disagreement over, for example, whether an operation should be performed or avoided. Now, however, they found themselves having to choose between practitioners who knew little or nothing about each other's fields, between practitioners who favored treating a wide array of illnesses with an approach derived from a single organizing concept – with each organizing concept seemingly unrelated to all the others.

How does one choose between, say, chiropractic, acupuncture, faith healing and nutrition? In fact, even if the choice is made to seek treatment from practitioners of one of these schools, how does one choose between practitioners who adhere to differing, and even opposing, movements within each school? It is hard enough to discover how competent and effective these practitioners are, let alone which ones to consult and in what order. The consumer is caught in a marketplace of competing claims, with nobody who is unbiased and knowledgeable enough to turn to for guidance.

Adrift and without a compass, decisions about treatment, which are some of the most important decisions in people's lives, are made in an unsystematic, haphazard manner. A practitioner is consulted because the next-door neighbor saw him and got better. Another is consulted because she makes fabulous (and unsubstantiated) claims. Still another is consulted because the clerk in the health foods store recommended him.

There is something to say for encouraging people to seek out forms of treatment that they believe in. Numerous studies have shown that, due to what has been labeled the placebo effect, people do better when they believe in the treatment. Despite the value of these placebo or non-specific effects, however, there are powerful specific effects of effective treatments which the consumer is entitled to receive. Furthermore, what about the dangers – physical, psychological and financial – of treatments rendered by unscrupulous and deluded practitioners who take advantage of their supplicants' plight, waste their time, expend their hope, and provide them with worthless remedies.

Recently, a third option has become increasingly available which makes it possible for people with treatment-resistant syndromes to continue in their search for symptom relief without having to abandon the relatively unbiased guidance of the medical practitioner. This option is Third Line Medicine. In contrast to other forms of medical specialization, the boundaries of third line medical practice are defined, not by the nature of the illness, but by the failure of the symptoms to respond to second line treatments. Third line physicians are not specialists in a particular disease or organ system; they are medical ecologists who seek to move their patients towards healing with treatments which reinforce natural adaptive mechanisms.

Third Line Medicine is defined as that portion of the practice of medicine which is devoted to improving the state of health of patients whose illnesses continue to cause distressing symptoms following standard courses of treatment by medical specialists. It extends the practice of medicine beyond its previous limits, just as the second line medical specialists extended medicine beyond the range of general practice. Since it caters to a specific patient population, it is a medical specialty – although it is a different form of specialty as it maintains a 'whole person' perspective which other specialties tend to lose.

Third Line Medicine is unique in its attempt to integrate the vast body of medical knowledge with methods of healing which utilize neither medicines nor surgery. It serves as a link between first and second line physicians, on the one hand, and alternative healing methods on the other. Third line physicians provide their patients with the guidance they need so that they, in partnership with all their treating physicians, can select appropriate treatments in a rational manner, treatments which can be provided concomitantly and/or sequentially according to the patients' needs.

In contrast to most non-medical practitioners, third line physicians maintain a strong commitment to scientific medicine. They attempt to keep abreast of the relevant scientific literature and continually incorporate new scientific findings into their methods of practice. Procedures which have greater scientific validation are chosen over procedures which appear to be equally appropriate, but lack proof of their efficacy. They temper their scientific knowledge, however, with their knowledge of the art of medicine, aware that much of the salutary effect of the treatment process has not, and perhaps cannot, be fully analyzed by science.

If, at times, they stray further from scientific practices than their second line colleagues, they do so for two reasons. First, they limit themselves to treatments which encourage the healing process. They shun 'heroic' treatments and attempt to avoid treatments with the potential for serious adverse effects. Thus the worst that can happen is that the patient will fail to benefit from the treatment because the treatment is ineffectual. (It should be noted that many or most patients may also fail to benefit from treatments which have been *proven* effective.) Second, the generally accepted treatments have already been rendered by second line physicians without success.

Second line Medicine, despite its impressive achievements, is riddled with large gaps between its many specialties. These gaps have developed because each specialty, as it developed, went off in its own direction without any attempt to coordinate with the specialties in related areas. The result is that many patients have illnesses which do not fit well within the confines of any established medical specialty. They have been the lost souls of modern medicine. In Third Line Medicine, they are finding physicians who are equipped to help them.

Yet another unique feature of Third Line Medicine is its integration of psychological and behavioral techniques with medical treatments. In so doing, it goes well beyond the territory usually staked out by psychiatry (a second line specialty). For example, third line physicians utilize these techniques with patients who have no mental illness and thus would not be appropriate for psychiatric treatment.

In summary, Third Line Medicine attempts to restore to medical practice the aspects of care which the current system neglects. It counters the compartmentalization of specialty care with an integrated approach; it restores the caring relationship between doctor and patient which technology has increasingly eroded; it restricts itself to uncommonly safe treatments; it introduces procedures which are so broad in their application that no single specialty claims them; it even introduces carefully selected procedures which, though safe, have yet to earn consensual validation in the medical community either because of inadequate scientific proof of their efficacy or because of unscientific bias against them.

Third Line Medicine is a growing movement, a movement which is unorganized and, up until now, unrecognized. It is a grassroots movement composed of practicing physicians who have expanded beyond their formal specialties in their desire to help their patients when they no longer have anywhere to go within the traditional system of medical practice. The movement is fueled, not by the need of these physicians to deny their impotence, but by their knowledge and experience which has taught them that many third line patients can indeed be helped.

In these pages, we shall undertake an exploration into the past and present world of western medicine in order to gain an appreciation of the roots from which Third Line Medicine has grown. (Although, for simplicity, we will concentrate on American medicine, the principles discussed are applicable in large measure to all western democratic societies.) We will focus on the deficiencies of the current system which cry out for correction. We shall examine the role of science in medicine, and the failure of the current system to incorporate present-day concepts of science into medical practice. Then we shall be ready to examine what I believe to be the basic principles of Third Line Medicine and its contribution to the treatment of illness in our society today.

It is my hope that this book will serve as an inspiration to both physicians and patients. The path towards health does not have to be abandoned when the established medical specialties can do no more; if patients wish to continue to fight for their health, and their doctors are willing to fight along with them, steps along the healing path may still be taken.

It would be tragic to abandon hope any earlier.

CHAPTER 2
Perils of the Hippocratic legacy

> I swear by Apollo Physician, by Asclepius, by Panacea and by all the gods and goddesses, making them my witnesses, that I will carry out, according to my ability and judgment, this oath and this indenture.

So begins an oath written twenty-five centuries ago and still repeated as a rite of passage when medical students become doctors of medicine. By taking this ancient oath, modern physicians acknowledge their historical allegiance to the teachings of an ancient Greek physician and teacher whose momentous contributions have earned him the title of Father of Western Medicine. His name was Hippocrates.

Who was this ancient Greek who laid the foundations for medicine as we know it today? We actually know very little about his life. The son of a physician himself, he was born at Cos about 460 BC and died between 377 and 359 BC, probably at Larissa in Thessaly. He traveled widely; he is known to have been to Thassos, Athens, Thrace and elsewhere. His many students included his two sons and his son-in-law. He founded the Hippocratic School of Medicine which became competitive with the temple school of Aesculapius which leaned towards magic and religion, and the philosophical school which was mainly theoretical. Many books have been attributed to him, although none has ever been proven to actually have been written by him. It is thought that these books, whether written by him or his disciples, originally formed the library of the Hippocratic School at Cos.

Health, according to Hippocrates, is the expression of a harmonious balance between the various components of man's nature, the environment and ways of life. Mind and body are so influenced by each other that one cannot be considered without the other. Health, i.e. a healthy mind in a healthy body, is achieved by governing daily life in accordance with natural laws, which ensures an equilibrium between the different forces of the organism and those of the environment. While the prevailing religious beliefs attributed organic disease to the will of the gods, Hippocrates attributed disease to a disturbance in the physical body. This disturbance, he believed, is caused either by something in the patient's external environment or by the patient's emotional state. Conversely, emotional disorders can be caused by the patient's physical state.

Hippocrates believed that there was a natural tendency towards self-healing. 'Nature is the physician of disease.' Patients can often heal themselves by employing the proper procedures, and thus they have considerable responsibility for their health. 'A wise man ought to realize that health is his most valuable possession and learn how to treat his illnesses by his own judgment.' Physicians aid their patients through their ability to suggest rational treatments for their particular illnesses. Patients may employ these same treatments without consulting with doctors, but their selection of the appropriate treatment is more due to chance than to science.

> When those who employ no doctors fall sick and then recover, they must know that their cure is due either to doing something or to not doing it. It may be fasting or eating a great deal, drinking largely or taking little fluid, bathing or not bathing, exercise or rest, sleep or wakefulness, or perhaps it is a mixture of several of these that is responsible for their cure.

Medicine, according to Hippocrates, is a science based on a fund of rational knowledge gained from careful observation. It is also an art ('of all the arts the most noble') which demands much of those who devote themselves to it. 'Life is short, and the Art long; the occasion fleeting; experience fallacious; and judgment difficult.' Only certain people should seek to become physicians. 'Whoever is to acquire a competent knowledge of medicine ought to be possessed of the following advantages: a natural disposition; instruction; a favorable position for the study; early tuition; love of labor; leisure.'

Hippocrates conceived the bailiwick of medicine as including all manner of objects present in the patients' environments as well as the manner in which they relate to these objects. Any and all of these objects may be utilized in the treatment, with safety a primary consideration. 'First do no harm.' 'Nothing should be omitted in an art which interests the whole world, one which may be beneficial to suffering humanity and which does not risk human life or comfort.' 'Not only must the physician be ready to do his duty, but the patient, the attendants and external circumstances must conduce to the cure.'

Procedures which foster natural healing are to be utilized as the first line of treatment. 'Leave your drugs in the chemist's pot if you can heal the patient with food.' Natural healing includes the therapeutic effects of a concerned and compassionate physician. 'Some patients, though their condition is perilous, recover their health simply through their contentment with the goodness of the physician.' Physicians must have 'kindly expressions' and avoid impatience with their patients if they wish to facilitate the healing process.

Through observation, Hippocrates developed a theory of the mechanism by which illness occurs. He recognized four different fluids or humors which circulate in the body – blood, phlegm, yellow bile and black bile – and postulated that, since these humors change in the course of illness, imbalances in the humors are the fundamental cause of both physical and mental illness. They, in turn, both influence and are influenced by the environment and the emotions. An excess of blood, for example, causes naive optimism, an excess of phlegm apathy, an excess of yellow bile anxiety and irritability and an excess of black bile sadness. The Hippocratic model of illness thus supposed that multiple factors may affect the genesis and resolution of the illness. Hippocrates argued for a systems approach in which both physical and psychosocial components of the complex ecosystem in which individuals exist could each contribute to their state of health. Physicians were not seen as merely scientists who delivered the correct treatments, but as important components of the ecosystem whose influence on the course of the illness was far more powerful than merely the biological effects of their specific remedies.

It was through the influence of Galen that Hippocrates' ecologic model was to survive for two thousand years. Galen (C. 130–220 AD), the greatest physician of Roman times, was a Greek physician who attended the Roman emperor Marcus Aurelius. Unlike Plato, who believed that matter was a slave to the spirit, Galen claimed that the soul was the slave to the body, since warmth, dampness, structure and animal spirits circulating in the body determined how one thought and felt. He was the first to claim that mental illness originated in the brain.

Galen's system of medicine incorporated the Hippocratic notion that humoral imbalances caused both physical and mental disorders. Delirium was thought to result from an excess of yellow bile in the brain, loss of memory and intelligence from an excess of phlegm or other cooling matter. Treatment of these diseases consisted of the elimination of the excess bile through phlebotomy or by the administration of cathartics.

Galen was well aware of the relationship between physical illness and the emotions. For example, he noted that psychic imbalance and anxiety could result from the retention of sperm in the male or the delay of uterine discharges in the female. He spoke of the correlation between hysterical symptoms and the absence of sexual relations and noted the curative effect of such relations.

The eventual fall of the Roman empire was followed by ten centuries (500–1500 AD) which are remarkable for their lack of scientific achievements. During these Middle or Dark Ages, with the Church the dominant force in western culture, religion and superstition returned to positions of prominence in the theory and practice of medicine. Disease was once again considered to be the result of sinful behavior or the work of witches and demons which required religious rituals for treatment.

Surprisingly, the influence of Galen continued throughout these many centuries, although the Galenic physicians rigidly adhered to their master's texts and added little to his contributions. Moses Maimonides (1135–1204 AD), a Jewish physician and a philosopher of Spanish origin, was a notable exception to the mixing of mysticism and medicine. Among his many contributions, he wrote in opposition to the use of magic and astrology and argued that there was a close relationship between a person's mental and physical health.

With the coming of the Renaissance (1500–1700 AD), the power of the Church began to ebb as science once again became a powerful force in western culture. It was a philosopher, René Descartes (1596–1650), who was to return the scientific study of the human body to a position of legitimacy. Descartes re-explored the ancient question of the relationship between the nature of the physical body and the ethereal realm of mind and spirit. His conclusion: both matter and spirit are real, with spirit preceding matter. Both meet and interact, he postulated, at the pineal gland.

Since mind was separate from body, physicians could study and treat the human body outside the pale of the Church. No longer was it heresy to investigate and treat natural causes of disease. Dramatic developments in mathematics, physics and chemistry could be utilized in the development of new tools for medical investigations, and the results of these investigations could be applied to medical practice.

Cartesian dualism freed the study and treatment of diseases of the body from the clutches of the Church; the mind, however, was left behind to remain for a few more centuries outside medicine and within the provinces of theology, philosophy and, eventually, 'romantic' (i.e. non-scientific) psychology. Renaissance medicine also signaled the decline in influence of the Galenic physicians. These physicians had managed to carry the torch of Hippocrates for fifteen centuries. Now advances in medical science began to invalidate their archaic humoral concepts, while their broad ecologic philosophy was increasingly eclipsed by the growing popularity of Cartesian dualism.

Despite the continuing restriction of medical practice to diseases of the body, the period of the seventeenth and eighteenth centuries was one of major advances in the tools and methods of scientific medicine. The invention of the microscope by Leeuwenhoek (1632–1723) enabled physicians to examine diseased tissues in a detail which had never before been possible. He also laid the groundwork for the germ theory of disease by being the first to observe the 'very tiny animalcules' which we now call bacteria and protozoa. Morgagni (1682–1771), by examining diseased tissues after death and correlating the patients' systems with the condition of their organs, proved that diseased organs caused illness. He thus discredited the humoral theory of Hippocrates and Galen.

It was not until the nineteenth century, however, that the humoral theory was dealt its fatal blow when Rudolph Virchow (1821–1902) traced the origin of disease to the cell. Through painstaking laboratory work, Virchow demonstrated that disease begins with a change toward pathology within living cells. A change in the structure of the cells is next to evolve, followed by the development of a physiological disorder of the cells that make up the tissue of the organ.

Perhaps the cornerstone of nineteenth century medicine was the development of the germ theory of infection which can be traced back to the French chemist Louis Pasteur (1822–95). In 1877, Pasteur observed that cultures of the bacteria responsible for anthrax lost their ability to cause disease when they became contaminated with microorganisms that lived in the soil and postulated that the contaminants produced a substance which neutralized them. This perceptive observation was to stimulate the development of what we now call antibiotics.

Science had now not only disproven Hippocrates' humoral theory of disease, but had proven that the presence of a microorganism was necessary for the development of certain diseases. Moreover, different diseases were associated with the presence of different microorganisms – each germ was specific for each disease – and the eradication of the microorganism cured the disease. These brilliant discoveries generated tremendous interest in the development of laboratory science in the hope that, in time, more and more diseases would be found to be associated with specific agents, agents which could then be eradicated with specific treatments.

This was a new way to view illness, as different from the ecologic model of Hippocrates as his model was different from the religious model. The late René Dubos, an esteemed microbiologist and Professor Emeritus at The Rockefeller University, has named this organizing paradigm *the doctrine of specific etiology*, and considers it to be the single most powerful force in the development of medicine in the past century (Dubos). Many other terms have been used: the biomedical model, the biological-reductionist model, the ontological model, the law of parsimony, etc.. None, however, conveys the central tenets of this paradigm as well as the name chosen by Dubos.

In essence, the doctrine has two major postulates:

1 Illness can be categorized into specific diseases.
2 Each disease has a unique primary cause.

The first postulate assumes that a disease is a real and distinct entity in nature rather than merely a label which serves as a convenient method of grouping a collection of signs and symptoms. Illness, it assumes, is simply the experience of being diseased. By implication, illnesses for which no specific disease can be discovered are less real than those with specific pathological changes. In addition, the non-specific aspects of illness (malaise, depression, etc.) do not require as much attention from the physician since they will disappear once the disease is treated successfully.

The second postulate assumes the existence of a specific agent for each disease. It further assumes that the agent whose presence is necessary for the existence of a disease is actually the cause of that disease. Other factors associated with a disease but neither specific to that disease nor necessary for its existence are considered to be irrelevant unless the specific etiologic agent has not yet been identified or cannot be eradicated.

This was an era in which infectious diseases were the major cause of death. The germ theory of disease, which served as the model for the doctrine of specific etiology, inspired the development of both antibiotics and immunization, introduction of which was followed by a rapid decline in the prevalence of fatal infections. Both the medical profession and the public credited the new medical treatments for causing the decline, and the development of medical investigation and practice based upon specific etiology doctrine became assured.

Beguiled by the dramatic results achieved through the introduction of antibiotics and immunization, people failed to recognize the evidence that most of the common infections had actually declined in incidence to a low level even before these treatments were introduced. Other factors, factors which were far more powerful in their impact upon public health, were also causing the decline. Thomas McKeown, Professor of Social Medicine Emeritus at the University of Birmingham in England, identifies these factors as 'the provision of food, protection from hazards, and limitation of numbers (McKeown). Malnutrition, lack of sewage and other protections from contamination with infectious agents, and overcrowding had fostered the transmission of infections and *their* correction was largely responsible for the conquest of fatal infections. Thus, while disregarded at the time, the ecologic model, since it takes all factors into consideration, provided a more powerful approach to the understanding and treatment of infectious diseases than did specific etiology doctrine.

With the development of the doctrine of specific etiology, and the abandonment of the humoral theory, the ecologic model fell into disrepute. The ecological model was never disproven; it simply appeared to be far simpler to pursue the 'magic bullet' than to have to deal with the complexities of a systems-oriented model. Instead of having to deal with the multitude of vaguely interrelated factors which impinged upon each individual's illness, researchers could now simplify their investigations by ignoring all but the unique aspects of each disease.

This dramatic change in the predominant medical model was accomplished without the necessity of devaluing Hippocrates. Since the Hippocratean corpus contains the writings of many physicians, it was riddled with internal inconsistencies. One group of writings, in fact, espouses a model which differs considerably from the rest of the corpus. While most of the works view the organism as an unanalyzable whole, these writings claim that the functioning of the organism and its relations with the environment are analyzable in terms of chains of causes progressing from external causes to internal ones, and ultimately to the production of symptoms. Medical diagnosis, therefore, aims to discover the cause of the disease; medical treatment seeks to oppose this cause by giving 'contrary' medicine (Coulter).

In the ninteenth century, when science was believed to be the knowledge of causes, these were the Hippocratic writings which were felt to be the truly scientific ones. Thus Hippocrates retained favor as the Father of Medicine even while the ecologic model, the model entertained in the greater body of Hippocratic writings, was relegated to the same fate as the antiquated humoral theory.

Despite the esteem for science, very little of the practice of medicine in that era was scientific. For example, the President of the Massachusetts Medical Society, speaking to his colleagues at their annual dinner meeting in 1858, concluded that:

> The cumbrous fabric now called therapeutic science is, in a great measure, built up on the imperfect testimony of credulous, hasty, prejudiced, or incompetent witnesses. . . . The enormous polypharmacy of modern times is an excredescence on science, unsupported by any evidence of necessity of fitness, and of which the more complicated formulas are so arbitrary and useless, that, if by any chance they should be forgotten, not one in a hundred of them would ever be reinvented. (Bigelow)

Even by the turn of the century, there was relatively little science in the practice of medicine. In the United States, for example, only 50 of the 155 medical schools were university-based, the rest being proprietary. The university schools, like Hopkins, Harvard and Yale, considered themselves to be superior to the proprietary schools and, indeed, they had better facilities and were unique in providing training in the scientific method. There was little evidence, however, that their training produced better practitioners (Brown).

The proprietary schools depended solely upon their students' fees for their existence. Since these fees were divided between the owners of the schools and the local practitioners who lectured there, little funding was left for technical facilities, such as laboratories and equipment. Faculty chairs were bought and sold, often at high prices, as they were looked upon as financial investments. Advertising was popular, since profits depended upon the number of students who could be convinced to enroll.

Medical education in these schools was based on the

apprenticeship model, with the curriculum designed to provide students with the empirical knowledge which the members of the faculty had acquired over their lifetimes in general practice. There was no outside control, so each school provided whatever curriculum it pleased. Students were accepted upon completing four years of high school or the 'equivalent'. Admission standards were low, courses were informal, and the quality of education was uneven at best.

Publication by the Carnegie Foundation in 1910 of *Medical Education in the United states and Canada* spelled the demise of the proprietary schools and thus ushered in the era of scientific medicine for these countries. Under the sponsorship of the Foundation, Abraham Flexner, the report's author, made a personal inspection of each medical school. The administrators and faculties, tempted by the prospect of receiving funding from Carnegie, and fearful of the adverse publicity which would be generated if they failed to cooperate, provided him with detailed information on every relevant aspect of their school's curricula, facilities, students and faculties.

In his report, Flexner argued that 'the country needs fewer and better doctors,' and 'the way to get them better is to produce fewer' (Flexner). He claimed that the proprietary schools kept the standard of medical education low, and believed that, in order to upgrade medical education and provide it with a modern scientific base, only the university schools should be permitted to remain. He proposed a minimal admission requirement of two years of college, even though only 5 per cent of the college age population was enrolled in a college at that time. In this manner, the social status and incomes of physicians would be raised to a level he deemed appropriate.

The changes Flexner proposed had already begun prior to the publication of his report, although the report was widely read and influential in accelerating the trend. Between 1904 and 1915, some ninety-two medical schools closed or merged, including schools which taught what would now be called 'alternative medicine' such as schools of homeopathy and schools whose orientations were eclectic. Extramural funding from foundations and governmental agencies became a major source of financing the cost of medical education. In contrast to earlier days when student fees were the sole source of funds, medical schools were denied extramural funds unless they adopted a research orientation, thus assuring that scientific medicine would be taught.

Through the impetus of the Flexner report, American and Canadian medicine now entered into the age of science. These countries were not alone, however, as similar changes were occurring almost simultaneously in other western nations. The transformation of medicine from an empirical to a scientific orientation was to lead to an explosion of knowledge unlike anything the world had previously known. The rigors of scientific methodology demanded that the practice of medicine would never again become frozen at a level of knowledge; there would be a constant input of new knowledge fed down from the research laboratories to the medical practitioners which would induce them continually to modify their practices.

Would Hippocrates have been proud? Undoubtedly he would have lauded the employment of more precise and replicable methods of scientific investigation. Modern scientific methods did not enter medicine, however, until after the doctrine of scientific etiology had supplanted Hippocrates' ecologic model. He would have seen that science was being applied, not to fill in the holes in our comprehension of the ecologic model, but to pursue reductionistic hypotheses seeking ultimate causes for multidetermined diseases.

Finally, he would have seen what the practice of medicine had become under the influence of specific etiology doctrine (which is exactly what we shall do in the next chapter). I believe he would have seen the folly of crediting the doctrine for medical progress which was due to other factors, and I believe he would have pleaded to modern physicians to return to the ecologic model and apply scientific methodology to increasing our knowledge within that model – before the yoke of the doctrine of specific etiology would bring the practice of medicine to a state of crisis from which it would be hardpressed to recover.

CHAPTER 3
Tarnish in the Golden Age

> Doctors are men who prescribe medicines of which they know little, to cure diseases of which they know less, in human beings of whom they know nothing.
>
> VOLTAIRE
> 1694–1778

Our society has made a massive commitment to the development and delivery of health care services, funding for which has been escalating so rapidly that, in recent years, increases in health care expenditures have usually exceeded increases in the gross national product (the market value for *all* goods and services produced by the economy) in both the United States and in most other industrialized nations (Ehrlich). Before 1950, less than one month's income was spent by the average American wage earner each year for the purchase of medical services; in the mid-1970s, the average wage earner was working for five to seven weeks to purchase them. In 1950, the United States spent $10 billion for health care; by 1985, health care expenditure had reached over $360 billion – about $1 billion dollars daily – and accounted for 11 per cent of the gross national product compared to only 4.4 per cent of the GNP a generation earlier.

While the United States has had the dubious distinction of far outdistancing the rest of the world in health care spending, other western nations have also been faced with mounting costs. Great Britain was estimated to have spent $400 dollars per person in 1984; Japan $500 per person; France $800 per person and West Germany $900 per person.

Technological developments are responsible for much of the massive increase in the cost of health care. A succession of increasingly sophisticated devices have provided methods of visualizing the depths of the human body without the need of a scalpel. X-rays, computerized axial tomography, diagnostic ultrasound and nuclear magnetic resonance scanning have each revolutionized the field of non-invasive somatic diagnosis, but have also carried a high price tag. Laboratory analyses of bodily fluids have also proliferated at a rapid rate, so that there are now about a thousand different tests available just for blood.

Diagnostic tests have become so central to the practice of medicine that over ten billion of these tests are currently being performed annually in the United States. The total bill for diagnostic testing has grown to be so enormous that it now amounts to about nearly half of the total cost of health care (Bechtel).

Not only has medical diagnosis become high-tech, but medical treatment has also become increasingly tied to the use of sophisticated and expensive devices. Radiation treatment for cancer and kidney dialysis are two common examples. The cost of care for the critically ill has skyrocketed as technological advances have spurred the development of elaborate intensive care units. We have entered the age of plastic man with the development of artificial bones and internal organs, but at an enormous price.

One would expect that the public's return on its investment in high technology medicine has justified the cost. Unfortunately, compared to the size of the investment, the benefits to the public from recent advances in medical diagnosis and treatment have been pitifully small. One critic, speaking at the First Conference on Electronics in Medicine, concluded that:

> most of the electronic devices and computerized systems that have been tried are sophisticated, unreliable, hard to use, and extremely expensive. There is little reason to believe, considering all their side effects, that they save the physician much time and effort. (Siebert)

Evidence for such a shocking statement comes from a recent Harvard study. When investigators compared the results of a hundred autopsies performed at their hospital in 1960, 1970 and 1980, they found that the percentage of diagnostic errors was about the same in each of the three eras (Goldman *et al.*).

They therefore failed to find evidence that modern diagnostic testing has actually improved medical diagnosis; yet physicians, complacent in their faith in these tests, have increasingly lost interest in performing post-mortum examinations. Since these examinations reveal disease which had been missed, they are an invaluable means of enhancing diagnostic skills. In the years after World War Two, the autopsy rate in the United States was 50 per cent. Since then there has been a progressive decline. As of 1973, it was down to 22 per cent as of 1983, it was down to barely 15 per cent. (Geller)

Further evidence for the rather meager benefits from diagnostic testing comes from a British study which examined the use of laboratory tests in the management of 174 emergency hospital admissions. Of all the routine blood and other biochemical tests ordered, only 2 per cent resulted in any change at all in treatment. According to the researchers:

> There can be little doubt that many tests are requested thoughtlessly. . . . It is difficult to avoid the conclusion that these investigations were a waste of resources. (*Annals of Clinical Biochemistry* November, 1980)

To be sure, life expectancy has shown a dramatic rise over the course of the century – due largely to decreased mortality during infancy and childhood (Arehart-Treichel). This was not, however, a victory of modern medicine. According to John H. Knowles, President of the Rockefeller Foundation,

> The marked increase in life expectancy at birth was due to the control and eradication of infectious disease, directly through improved nutrition and personal hygiene, and environmental changes, namely, the provision for safe water and milk supplies and for sewage disposal. (Knowles)

Adds Jacob Brody, Associate Director at the National Institute on Aging,

> It wasn't doctors who were so much responsible for [improved sanitation, although] they like to take credit for it. But I suspect that the man who invented screens did more. Certainly the man who invented the flush toilet did more. (op. cit.)

Lewis Thomas, President of the Memorial Sloan-Kettering Cancer Center, has surveyed medical progress in the third quarter of this century. His conclusions:

> The most spectacular technological change has occurred in the management of infectious disease, but its essential features had been solidly established and put to use well before 1950. . . . There has been no quantum leap in anti-infectious technology since 1950. Several new virus vaccines have been developed. The antibiotics have come into more widespread use . . . ; a multiplicity of new variants of antibiotics and chemotherapeutic agents have appeared on the market. . . . There have been a few other examples of technology improvement, comparable in decisive effectiveness, since 1950, but the best of these have been for relatively uncommon illnesses. . . . We are left with approximately the same roster of common major diseases which confronted the country in 1950, and, although we have accumulated a formidable body of information about some of them in the intervening time, the accumulation is not yet sufficient to permit either the prevention or the outright cure of any of them. (Thomas, 1977)

Cardiovascular disease is the leading cause of death, with roughly one million Americans dying annually of heart disorders or strokes (Trafford). As of 1985, Americans were paying seventy-two billion dollars annually for the treatment of heart disease alone – up from four billion in 1971. One and a half million Americans were predicted to suffer a heart attack during the year, with over half a million predicted to die from the attack (*Heart Facts*).

Few people realize that coronary arteriosclerosis, the major cause of cardiovascular death, is a disease of the twentieth century. It was unrecognized before 1890 (Zucker) and was virtually unknown until sixty or seventy years ago (Bradshaw). While American soldiers killed in World War One and subsequently autopsied were rarely found to have cardiovascular disease, in the Vietnam War it was rare to find a soldier whose body did not show evidence of the disease. (op. cit.)

Despite the numerous research projects seeking to identify

the pathologic events which cause arteriosclerosis, they remain largely unknown. Adequate technological interventions have yet to be found to prevent the disease from developing. With the exception of surgery for congenital heart disease, we are unable to cure cardiovascular diseases once they become established (Thomas, 1977).

There is some good news. Cardiovascular mortality has been declining in the United States since 1968. According to the Department of Health and Human Services of the United States government, deaths from heart disease declined by 39 per cent between 1950 and 1983, while deaths from strokes plummeted by 48 per cent. This decline, however, does not appear to be attributable to increased spending on medical care or to technological advances. Rather it appears to be due to increasing public awareness about the dangers of certain behaviors such as smoking, excessive fat consumption and the lack of exercise (Stamler, Kannel).

Cancer is the second leading cause of death from disease. In 1971, the National Cancer Act was passed in the United States as President Nixon and Congress declared 'war on cancer' and the budget of the National Cancer Institute was increased from $180 million to more than $1 billion annually. There have been limited areas of substantial progress since then. For example, patients with once-fatal disorders such as Hodgkin's Disease and certain childhood leukemias now have a better than 50 per cent chance for long-term survival. Yet, since the 'war' was declared, the chances of an American contracting cancer have risen from 1 in 6 to nearly 1 in 3! While people born in 1950 had a 19 per cent probability of developing cancer by age eighty-five, people born in 1981 had a 27 per cent risk of developing cancer by that age (Epstein).

Although 44 per cent of the $1 billion dollar budget of the National Cancer Institute goes toward basic research, a fundamental understanding of the causes of cancer remains decades away. We have yet to develop a method of eliminating the biological processes which transform normal cells into malignant ones and we are unable to reverse the neoplastic process once it begins (Thomas, 1977).

According to the National Diabetes Commission, diabetes mellitus is the third leading cause of death in the United States, accounting for a third of a million deaths annually. The American Diabetes Association estimates that one out of twenty people will be diabetic sometime in the course of their lifetime. By contrast, not long ago diabetes was a rare disease; its prevalence has risen *600 per cent* from 1935 to 1978! Specific etiologists are at a loss to account for the dramatic increase of diabetes in the population. It has been attributed to the increased lifespan, but since the increase in lifespan is largely due to decreased mortality among the newborn, it can hardly explain the bulk of the rise.

The discovery of insulin has been a major step forward. Insulin deficiency, however, can hardly be the underlying cause of all diabetic complications, since the vascular disease proceeds even when supplemental insulin is regularly provided. While we can now prevent death from diabetic coma, we still know almost nothing about the vascular disease which kills by causing kidney failure, heart attacks and strokes, and we have no new treatment to stop its progression (Thomas, 1977).

Considering that Americans spend more money on health care and have more doctors than citizens of any other country, it is shocking to find that men living in fourteen other countries have a greater life expectency than American men, while women in six other countries have a greater life expectancy than American women. Sweden has the lowest infant mortality rate in the world, while the United States has one of the highest of any industrial nation. Frank Chappell, a spokesperson for the American Medical Association, claims that international health statistics are misleading:

> In the U.S. there is a huge mix of all races and backgrounds. Comparing a country like Sweden, which has one of the highest life expectancies, with the United States, is like comparing apples and oranges. If you compared Swedes from Minnesota to Swedes from Sweden, the Minnesota Swedes live longer. (Bricklin)

It just so happens that such a study has been completed, and the results have been published in the *American Journal of Public Health*. The author, Richard F. Tomasson, Ph.D. of the University of New Mexico, compared death rates for Swedish men with those of male caucasians living in Minnesota (where the geography, economy and country of ancestry resemble conditions in Sweden) and found that Americans are dying at a faster rate at each and every age bracket throughout life until the age of eighty. Even when Swedish men are compared to white men living in Utah, which has one of the lowest white male mortality rates in the country, Swedish men live longer. For example, a white male between the ages of fifty and fifty-four in Utah has a 45 per cent greater chance of dying than a white male of the same age in Sweden (Tomasson).

The obvious question is why, despite the impressive achievements in the development of highly sophisticated tools for diagnosis and treatment, has modern American medicine achieved so little in the understanding and conquest of illness? The answer, I suggest, lies not in the tools of medicine, but in the devotion of modern American physicians to the doctrine of specific etiology. Gone is the ecologic model espoused by Hippocrates; instead modern physicians narrow their vision to employ specific treatments for supposedly specific diseases. Gone is adherence to Hippocrates' dictum of 'first do no harm'; instead, modern physicians act as if the more powerful the intervention, the better the outcome – as if they were in a battle with a foreign invader. Since patients provide the battleground, they are encouraged to agree to dangerous but powerful treatments as the procedures of choice. Only when these treatments have failed do they suggest treatments which encourage self-healing, as if these more natural treatments were far less powerful than the dangerous ones.

Thomas McKeown, Professor of Social Medicine Emeritus at the University of Birmingham in England, is convinced that:

> Doctors have always tended to overestimate the effectiveness of their intervention and to underestimate the risks, whether removing large quantities of blood, under mistaken notions of the blood volume, in the treatment of yellow fever in the eighteenth century, or exposing patients to dangerous levels of radiation, of whose effects they were unaware, when screening for breast cancer in the twentieth. (McKeown)

These risks are formidable. According to Ivan Illich:

> The pain, dysfunction, disability, and anguish resulting from technical medical intervention now rival the morbidity due to traffic and industrial accidents and even war-related activities, and make the impact of medicine one of the most rapidly spreading epidemics of our time. Among murderous institutional torts, only modern malnutrition injures more people than iatrogenic disease in its various manifestations. (Illich)

Iatrogenic illness, illness created by physician's interventions, has indeed become a problem of massive proportions. Before the modern era, iatrogenic illness was essentially a problem of medical treatment; now it is also a problem arising from medical diagnostic interventions. Our sophisticated diagnostic equipment is often capable of causing illness – and even death – but modern physicians, enamored of the gadgetry and fiercely dedicated to establishing a specific diagnosis, tend to overutilize it and underestimate its potential destructiveness. Just diagnostic x-rays alone have been estimated by experts to cause thousands of cancers and leukemias, resulting in between 3,500 and 30,000 deaths annually (Freese).

Medications are now so much a part of our lifestyle that, every twenty-four to thirty-six hours, from 50 to 80 per cent of adults in the United States are believed to swallow a medically prescribed chemical (Illich). Adverse reactions to these medications result in roughly 1.5 million patient visits to doctors' offices and hospitals annually (Freese), and 3 per cent of hospital admissions are due to drug reactions. The ten million people hospitalized in medical units of hospitals annually receive an average of nine courses of drug therapy each. This results in six million immediate adverse reactions and an unknown amount of adverse reactions due to delayed and long-term effects. Of this group, 29,000 people, about one in 340, die each year as a result of the reaction (Jick). They constitute about half of the 60,000 people who die each year in the United States because of adverse reactions to drugs (Talley and Laventurier).

The greater the number of medications prescribed for a patient, the greater the chance of adverse effects due to interactions between the drugs and errors in administering them. One computer study found that 84 per cent of a group of 42,000 Californians were given combinations of drugs which presented serious problems of interactions (Freese). Other studies have shown that an error in the administration of medications ordered by the physicians occurs once in every six or seven dosages administered on a hospital ward (Cook).

Even the experts cannot protect the public from adverse reactions to medications which are unknown at the time these medications are prescribed. Strict governmental standards requiring scientific proof of the safety and efficacy of new drugs have repeatedly failed to prevent the eventual relabeling or removal of medications from the market after they had been released as additional adverse effects became apparent. Examples are all too numerous. Sleeping pills and minor tranquilizers had been marketed for years before their addictive potential was recognized. The birth control pills had become extremely popular before it was discovered that they may cause serious, and even lethal, cardiovascular side effects, and the carcinogenic effects of post-menopausal estrogen replacement therapy became known years after its employment had become popular.

Despite their potential for adverse side effects, there remain, of course, many situations in which the use of medications is the appropriate form of treatment. As an article in *The New England Journal of Medicine* points out:

> The benefit-to-risk ratio for the vast majority of commonly used drugs appears to be a reasonable one justifying the proper use of these drugs. . . . The large number of hospitalizations resulting from adverse drug reactions is a reflection more of the vast usage of drugs than of their toxicity. . . . Thus, if we wish to reduce the amounts of drug toxicity substantially we must reduce the number of drugs that people take. (Jick)

Unfortunately, the evidence is that, even if we exclude the use of alternative treatments, a significant portion of that vast usage of drugs is due to the tendency of physicians to overprescribe. James A. Visconti, Director of the Drug Information Center at Ohio State University, claims that three-quarters of the adverse reactions to drugs are predictable, and most could be prevented without losing their beneficial effects if physicians would use them more rationally (Freese). David C. Lewis, a professor at Harvard Medical School, surveyed Boston physicians and found that two-thirds of them agreed that doctors prescribe too many sedatives, tranquilizers and amphetamines (ibid.).

Antibiotics are one of the classes of drugs which are overprescribed. Penicillin alone causes reactions in 9 to 10 per cent of patients and takes 100 to 300 lives annually in the United States; yet the United States Center for Disease Control, in a study of prescribing practices in seven community hospitals, found that antibiotics were being given to about one-third of all patients, even though nearly two-thirds of them had *no* documented infections! Other studies have found that between one-half to two-thirds of all prescriptions for anti-microbial drugs were irrational (ibid., Holmberg and Faich).

In their battle against disease, modern physicians concentrate upon prescribing such potent, and often dangerous, medications, while they neglect other forms of intervention which, besides being safer, are often more effective in reinforcing self-healing mechanisms. Roger Williams, the discoverer of pantothenic and folic acids (parts of the vitamin B complex), warns that:

> The basic fault of [drugs] is that they have no known connection with the disease process itself. . . . Drugs are wholly unlike nature's weapons. . . . They tend to mask the difficulty, not eliminate it. They contaminate the internal environment [with side effects], create dependence on the part of the patient, and often complicate the physician's job by erasing valuable clues as to the real source of the trouble. (Williams)

Much of the problem can be attributed to the belief of most practicing physicians that their prescribing decisions are made purely on objective, scientific grounds. John P. Morgan, Associate Professor of Medicine and Pharmacology at Mount Sinai School of Medicine, argues, however, that such a belief is naïve, and notes that 'prescribing is a complex psychosocial as well as medical event that is influenced by a variety of complex nonclinical and clinical factors. Physicians are often not as conscious of the psychological, social, and legal forces impinging upon the act of prescribing.' (Morgan) According to Doctor Morgan, physicians fail to consciously recognize and deal with the non-clinical factors which influence their prescribing practices because 'medical students as well as physicians engaging in postgraduate education programs are taught about drugs almost solely from a biological – reductionist viewpoint.' (ibid.)

In the United States, the multi-billion dollar pharmaceutical industry, well aware of physicians' naivete regarding their prescribing decisions, spends an estimated two billion dollars in order to advertise its wares to physicians (Jacobs). Thirty per cent of this staggering sum is spent on advertisements appearing in medical journals (Mckinley). The rest is spent on an army of 'detail men' who appear periodically in physicians' waiting rooms. These salespeople are especially trained to be knowledgeable about the scientific studies which validate their company's products and to promote the advantages of these products while appearing to be unbiased. Their approach is to seduce the doctor to prescribe their products due to their respectful demeanor, their 'scientific' knowledge, and their graciousness in providing free samples of the products they are pushing.

A Harvard University study has shown that physicians will pick up erroneous information from detail men, information which clearly is at variance with the scientific literature, and utilize that information in making decisions about prescribing (Avorn *et al.*). Milton Silverman, a member of the faculty at the University of California, San Francisco, laments that:

> In medical school, we teach students to prescribe on the basis of scientific evidence. . . . Five years after medical school, they are not prescribing as they were taught. They are brainwashed by detailers. (Jacobs)

If the doctrine of specific etiology is the contemporary religion of western medicine, then the modern hospital has become its house of worship. The hospital represents the pinnacle of high technologic, disease-oriented medical practices; thus it is modern medicine at its best. As such, it is also a monument to the tragic flaws of the doctrine which favors impersonal and unphysiologic procedures over procedures which attempt to rebalance the ill from an ecologic perspective. It is certainly not a place for a sick person; even a healthy person would be worn down by the authoritarian atmosphere with its often callous disregard for personal feelings and frequent, usually unnecessary, interruptions to sleep.

It is so dangerous a setting that hospital accidents are more frequent than accidents in all industries except mining and high-rise construction, with each patient risking a 7 per cent chance of suffering a compensatable injury (Illich). One of these risks is accidental electrocution due to malfunctioning electronic equipment, an event which occurs to an estimated 5,000 to 15,000 patients annually (Freese).

One out of every five patients admitted to a typical American research hospital acquires an iatrogenic disease which, in one case in thirty, leads to death (Illich). The *Journal of the American Medical Association* has published the results of a survey in which the authors studied all patients admitted to a hospital's intensive care unit over the course of one year. They found that one out of eight were hospitalized because of iatrogenic disease, and that almost half of these admissions were due to therapeutic or technical errors that were potentially avoidable (Trunet *et al.*).

Perhaps one out of every six patients acquires an infection from germs present on their ward. According to a magazine published by Blue Cross, there could be as many as 100,000 deaths annually in American hospitals due to such infections (Freese).

The fact that being in a hospital is not only inconvenient and uncomfortable, but also potentially dangerous, makes it all the more imperative that hospitalization be avoided in so far as is possible. Unfortunately, modern physicians overutilize it to such an extent that, in the United States, utilization review committees have been mandated by the Government to attempt to minimize unnecessary hospital stays. An example is the modern fashion of hospitalizing cardiac patients with acute illness in sophisticated and expensive coronary care units, which has failed to prove its value. A study reported in *The Lancet*, for example, failed to demonstrate any advantage of the coronary care unit over home care (Hill *et al*). In another study published in the *British Medical Journal*, the authors randomly picked persons with uncomplicated myocardial infarctions and sent them either to a coronary care unit or home to bed. They found that the mortality rate of patients sent to the CCU was actually *higher* than that of those sent home (Mather *et al.*)!

Almost half of the patients admitted into a hospital undergo surgery. Of all approaches to treatment, surgery may well be the ultimate one for the dedicated specific etiologist. If we are no more than a collection of interconnected parts, a part which malfunctions (i.e. becomes diseased) should ideally be removed and even replaced. The fact that surgery is expensive, disruptive to a patient's life, and carries an inherent risk of serious adverse effects, does little to temper its popularity compared to less invasive forms of treatment.

Our society has become so enamored of the act of surgery that it rewards physicians with considerably more money for operating on patients than for any other professional activity. Not only is surgery inherently dangerous with an overall mortality rate of 1.2 per cent, but surgical procedures are frequently performed even when the scientific evidence for their efficacy has yet to be established. The authors of an article in *Science* note that:

> New surgical operations may or may not be tested in animals, may be introduced as human therapy with or without review by a human experimentation committee and with or without a formal experimental design, and may or may not be evaluated by long-term follow-up observation. (Bunker *et al.*)

The result is that numerous operative procedures have suddenly become fashionable prior to being subjected to scientific investigation to evaluate if they were more effective and/or less dangerous than the procedures they replaced. Only later, after hundreds of people were put under the knife, many never to recover fully from the damage caused by the surgery, were these procedures found to be valueless and abandoned. These have included gastric freezing for peptic ulcer, colectomy for epilepsy, bilateral hypogastric artery ligation for pelvic hemorrhage, renal capsule stripping for acute renal failure, sympathectomy for asthma, internal mammary artery ligation for coronary artery disease, the 'button' operation for ascites, adrenalectomy for essential hypertension, complete dental extraction for 'focal sepsis', lobotomy for mental disorders, and wiring for aortic aneurysm (Hiatt).

A team of three Harvard physicians at the Office of Information Technology has reported on the eventual outcome of forty-six 'breakthroughs' in surgery or anesthesia which had been introduced into practice but only later had been critically evaluated. The authors concluded that only 13 per cent of these innovations proved to be 'highly preferred': about half of them (49 per cent) were only 'successful'. Twelve per cent were found to actually increase complications (Gilbert *et al.*). The current surgical procedure which leads all others in the cost of equipment, personnel, hospital space and total associated revenues is coronary bypass surgery. Introduced in 1967, the operation quickly became popular. Its rationale was simple: since the pain and mortality of coronary artery disease was due to blockage of the arteries which feed the heart, bypassing the blockage with grafts would restore the circulation to normal and would thus stop the pain and prolong life. By 1969, the operation was being performed at most of the nation's leading medical centers. Scientific studies were rejected as unnecessary, and cardiovascular surgeons refused on ethical grounds to withhold surgery from some patients so that comparative studies could be made (Preston).

By 1984, the procedure had become the established treatment for patients with severe 'stable' angina and occlusive disease involving at least two of the three major coronary arteries (Bunker *et al.*). About 200,000 Americans were undergoing bypass surgery annually at a cost of at least $25,000 each.

What has been the scientific evaluation of this procedure since its introduction two decades ago? Only six years before coronary bypass surgery was introduced, H. K. Beecher showed that the placebo effect could explain the benefits following surgery for angina pectoris due to coronary arteriosclerosis. He performed ligation of the internal mammary artery – the fashionable procedure of that day – on a group of angina patients. The operation reduced pain by 60 to 90 per cent and, according to the electrocardiogram, improved cardiac function. He then told a second group of patients he was going to perform the same procedure. Although he operated upon them, he performed a sham procedure and left the internal mammary artery alone. When the two groups were compared, he found that the second group benefited just as much as did the first (Beecher)!

Despite Beecher's study, since coronary bypass surgery was introduced, no studies have been undertaken to discover whether the relief of anginal pain is actually due to the grafts, or is once again merely a placebo effect. Furthermore, it is highly unlikely that such studies will *ever* be performed, since hospital human use committees will no longer permit sham operations to be performed for 'ethical' reasons.

A decade after the operation was introduced, studies which investigated the claim that coronary bypass surgery prolongs life finally began to be published – and lent little support to that claim. A 1977 United States Veterans Administration study showed that bypass surgery failed to decrease average annual mortality among patients with ordinary angina unless they had an obstructed left main coronary artery, while a 1978 National Institutes of Health study failed to find that bypass surgery was followed by a difference in survival rates for patients with unstable angina (Preston). Consistent with these findings were two more recent studies which failed to find a decrease in later heart attacks among patients who received bypass surgery after suffering one (ibid.).

Thomas Preston, Professor of Medicine at the University of Washington in Seattle, has stated that, as of 1985, the growing scientific literature suggests that bypass surgery is in large part only a placebo, and that fully half of the bypass operations performed in the United States are unnecessary. According to Doctor Preston, the literature suggests that only about 11 per cent of all bypass operations are performed on heart patients for whom surgery clearly prolongs life; another 10 per cent might have some extension of life owing to surgery – although we will have to wait several more years before studies tell us if this figure is too optimistic (ibid.).

When one considers the enormous expense of the operation, the tremendous emotional stress it imposes on patients and their families, and the chance of adverse complications, it is tragic that the scientific validation of coronary bypass surgery, just like the validation of other innovative surgical procedures, is so meager and so long in coming – while the acceptance of the procedure by the medical community was so hasty and uncritical.

Even worse than the frequent utilization of unproven operations is the performance of operations which have been proven to be valueless. There are perhaps as many as twenty million operations performed annually in the United States. A subcommittee of the House of Representatives concluded that, in 1974, 2.4 million of these procedures were unnecessary. These unnecessary procedures had resulted in 11,900 deaths and had cost four billion dollars (House of Representatives).

The most common surgical procedure in the United States is a tonsillectomy, with one million performed annually; yet, according to A. Frederick North, Jr., Visiting Professor of Pediatrics at the University of Pittsburgh, 90 to 95 per cent of these procedures are entirely unnecessary (*Christian Science Monitor* 138:98). In fact, reviews of the scientific data have concluded that there is no compelling evidence of long-term benefits from the operation (Evans, Paradise). Similarly, radical mastectomy is the most widely used operation for breast cancer even though there is strong evidence that it is no more effective in prolonging life and relieving symptoms than simpler procedures (Snyder). 3.5 million elective hysterectomies were performed on women of childbearing age in the United States between 1970 and 1979. Of this number, the Center for Disease Control has concluded that at least one of every seven had a 'questionable' indication since the patients' conditions were treatable by less drastic means (*Medical World News* 7 December 1981).

In addition to the risk of serious adverse effects, surgery as a treatment is subject to the danger of error on the part of the surgeon. Authors of a Harvard study found that general surgeons clearly violated basic surgical principles in about 1 per cent of cases, adding an average of $40,000 to the cost of treatment to each case. Of thirty-six surgical patients whose illnesses were complicated by surgical misjudgment, the errors contributed to the death of eleven, and seriously impaired the health of five more. Errors were due to misplaced optimism, unwarranted urgency, the urge for perfection and the desire to use 'new stylish procedures that have prestigious appeal.' (Couch *et al.*)

Despite their traditional rǫle of providing support for physicians, even some nurses are personally convinced that surgery is performed too readily. A recent survey by *RN*, the American national journal for nurses, found that one out of four nurses surveyed believed that between 30 and 49 per cent of all operations were unnecessary, while another fifth of the nurses claimed that the majority of operations were needless. 83 per cent of the nurses were willing to risk their jobs in order to tell patients of non-surgical alternatives to treatment, even if the doctor refused to do so (*Prevention* January 1982).

While practicing physicians are fast to employ the latest methods of diagnostic testing, drug therapy and surgery, they are woefully ignorant of the literature on alternative methods of diagnosis and treatment. An example is their naivete regarding the science of nutrition – which is an avenue of diagnosis and treatment so relevant to the clinical course of *all* illness that specific etiologists prefer to ignore it. Jean Mayer, President of Tufts University and an internationally acclaimed authority on nutrition, comments that his studies of Harvard physicians during specialty training 'suggest that the average physician knows a little more about nutrition than the average secretary – unless the secretary has a weight problem, and then she probably knows more than the average physician.' (Mayer) 'The area of nutrition has been neglected by the medical profession,' is the opening sentence of a recent commentary published in the *Journal of the American Medical Association*:

> Most medical schools devote less than three hours of total instruction to nutritional deficiency and therapy. Only 3 per cent of all questions on parts I, II, and III of the National Boards deal with the nutritional aspects of disease. In short, physicians in the United States are not required to have any understanding of nutrition to be licensed to practice medicine. (Wright)

It is therefore not surprising to find 'scientific' physicians ignoring nutritional factors as long as patients do not present with advanced symptoms of the classic vitamin deficiency diseases (Krehl). If nutritional factors in illness were indeed limited to gross starvation and the classical vitamin deficiency diseases, the failure to do a careful nutritional evaluation would be of minor importance. This, however, is not the case; what we ingest has a profound influence upon our state of health.

Roger J. Williams writes in *Nutrition Against Disease*:

> . . . the thesis is that *the nutritional microenvironment of any body cells is crucially important to our health and that deficiencies in this environment constitute a major cause of disease.*
>
> In cases of scurvy, pellagra, beriberi, or kwashiorkor, no physician would be inclined to question that the cause of the respective disease lies in the deficient microenvironment of the cells involved; but in orthodox medicine physicians are taught to think of this as a restrictive principle and to assume that the majority of illnesses with which they deal have virtually no connection with nutrition at all.
>
> Is this restrictive attitude really warranted? There is little evidence to support such restrictions and much evidence in favor of a wide extension of the nutritional approach to medicine. It is my opinion that medical theory, medical education, and medical practice have taken a wrong turn, and that all of us are the worse for it. (Williams)

This neglect has caused malnutrition to reach epidemic proportions in American hospitals (Rudman). Incredible as it may seem, over half the people in the medical wards of public and private hospitals in the United States are at various states of starvation (Butterworth, Wright). About half of the patients receiving surgery are also malnourished, even though malnutrition is well known to impair their chances for recovery from their operations (Mullen *et al.*, Thompson *et al.*). In the largest study to date, the nutritional status of over 3,000 patients in thirty-three hospitals was surveyed and 58 per cent were found to be malnourished. Only one out of three patients could even be surveyed, as the hospital staffs had not even bothered to perform basic nutritional screening on the majority of their patients. This is despite the well-established facts that malnutrition is associated with such factors as increased length of hospitalization, higher rates of infection, and poorer wound healing (*AMA News* May 24/31, 1985).

Hospital diets, rather than being designed to bolster the nutritional status of patients, may even contribute to the deficiencies. For example, researchers at the US Department of Agriculture's Human Nutrition Laboratory measured the amount of copper and zinc, both essential trace minerals, in hospital meals and found both to be significantly below the basic requirements for the average person in good health (Klevey *et al.*). A survey of patients in French hospitals has shown that this problem is not limited to the United States, as about half of the patients were receiving less than the Recommended Dietary Allowances for vitamins B1, B2 and B6 (Lemoine *et al.*).

The worst of all hospital diets is given to some of the sickest patients, namely those who are unable to take foods by mouth and thus must receive all their nutrition through intravenous feedings. As a recent article in the *Journal of the American Medical Association* points out, these patients may die of starvation due to lack of protein rather than of the illness which caused their hospitalization (Steffee). In addition, unless essential nutrients are added to their I.V. solutions (and they may not be!) they will develop severe deficiencies of macronutrients within one week (Chipponi *et al.*).

The marked contrast between their eager and uncritical utilization of unvalidated surgical procedures (no surgeon will ever be called a quack for doing coronary bypass grafts) and their marked skepticism for a form of treatment which reinforces the body's own regulatory mechanisms – even when there is considerable scientific validation for it – proves that the specific etiologists embrace science tightly when it advances their interests, but relax their grips when it does not.

Nowhere in contemporary medical practice is the abandonment of ancient healing principles by modern physicians so obvious as in their retreat from dealing with the human problems of their patients. Their neglect of the person while treating the disease is considered acceptable – and even cost-effective – in a medical world which subscribes to specific etiology doctrine. Writing in the *Journal of Clinical Psychiatry*, Robert R. Rynearson warns that:

> Increasing technology in medicine is pushing the physician away from the patient. If the physician allows machinery to be interposed between him and the patient, he will be in danger of forfeiting powerful healing influences. . . . Physicians must resist the idea that technology will some day abolish disease. As long as humans feel threatened and helpless, they will seek the sanctuary that illness provides. (Rynearson)

Patients have become keenly aware of the increasing distance modern medicine is placing between them and their doctors, and that their doctors are willing collaborators in the process. Nowhere has this process of alienation proceeded quite so far as in the United States. A recent American Medical Association survey, for example, reported that 60 per cent of patients think doctors are too interested in making money, while a Harris poll found that only 35 per cent of patients are satisfied with doctors in general (White). After reviewing studies of current public opinion, an article in the *Journal of Communication* concluded that:

> expressions of dissatisfaction with medical care have grown in volume and reflect a basic sense of confusion and frustration with the health care system on the part of the general population. (Daly and Hulka)

The National Citizens' Board on Inquiry into Health in America, with half of its members either physicians or leaders in the health care field, has studied the situation of the medical consumer and reached a similar conclusion:

> Unless one has faced a room of angry consumers . . . one cannot realize the extent or depth of that anger and frustration. . . . Let there be no mistake. The anger is well founded. The deficiencies are real. (Freese)

Angry patients have increasingly sought retribution against their doctors by taking them to court. In 1976, *Medical Economics* found that 8 per cent of patients in the United States had considered suing a doctor. By 1982, that percentage had risen to 13 per cent (Brown). By 1983, the annual number of malpractice claims had risen to a national average of eight claims per hundred physicians (Trubo)!

According to attorney Louise Lander, the increasing prevalence of malpractice litigation in the United States cannot be attributed to a rise in the commission of acts of malpractice so much as it is a consequence of the rising anger of patients towards physicians. The author of *Defective Medicine: Risk, Anger and the Malpractice Crisis*, she notes in her book that malpractice suits have two components: an injury *and* an angry patient. Patients sue, not merely because they believe that their doctors have acted improperly, but also because their doctors have alienated them (Lander).

Physicians, in turn, have tended to react to the public's alienation by alienating themselves still further. Witness the question a group of orthopedic surgeons posed to *Medical Economics*:

> We're sometimes asked for appointments by people who complain – either when they're calling for an appointment or during the first visit – about unsatisfactory treatment by other physicians. Since these patients seem like potential malpractice risks, we'd rather not get involved with them. Will we get into trouble if we refuse to accept them as patients? (*Medical Economics* 15 March 1982)

Physicians such as these are unconcerned with the possibility that patients who complain may have a legitimate grievance. Rather than attempt to show these patients that there are physicians who give good care, their concern is to protect themselves by denying care. Little do they realize that, by further alienating patients, they may avoid one malpractice suit but yet increase the overall risk of future suits against physicians.

Something, then, is clearly wrong, something which the infusion of massive governmental and private funds into health care delivery has been unable to correct. According to Aaron Wildavsky, President of the Russel Sage Foundation:

> Everyone knows that doctors do help. They can mend broken bones, stop infections with drugs, operate successfully on swollen appendices. Innoculations, internal infections, and external repairs are other good reasons for keeping doctors, drugs, and hospitals around. More of the same, however, is counterproductive. Nobody needs un-

> necessary operations; and excessive use of drugs can create dependence or allergic reactions or merely enrich the nation's urine. More money alone, then, cannot cure old complaints. In the absence of medical knowledge gained through new research, or of administrative knowledge to convert common practice into best practice, current medicine has gone as far as it can. It will not burn brighter if more money is poured on it. No one is saying that medicine is good for nothing, only that it is not good for everything. Thus the marginal value of one – or one billion – dollars spent on medical care will be close to zero in improving health. (Wildavsky)

Wildavsky, then, suggests that the quality of medical care cannot be enhanced by merely contributing more money to the current system. More knowledge, he says, must first be gained, either through medical research or through the development of 'administrative knowledge'. Progress in both these areas, however, has been thwarted by the domination of the doctrine of specific etiology.

Despite the disappointing benefits to health from the many thousands of research studies pursuing specific etiologies, apologists continue to maintain that, if only we maintain our pursuit long enough, it will eventually pay off. Both Lewis Thomas, for example, President of the Memorial Sloan-Kettering Cancer Center, and Ivan Bennett, Jr., Dean of the New York University School of Medicine, believe that we are in the midst of an era of 'half-way technologies' which consist of measures designed to palliate the manifestations of diseases we remain unable to prevent or cure – such as organ transplants and kidney dialysis. While they admit that such current procedures are extremely expensive, Thomas and Bennett believe that their high costs are only temporary since research will eventually unlock the secrets of the diseases for whose treatment these procedures were developed. They cite examples of diseases whose treatments were expensive only until their specific etiologies were discovered to back up their contention that prevention and cure of the diseases which currently plague our society will also become possible and relatively inexpensive once their root causes are found (Bennett, Thomas, 1974).

One cannot argue against promoting medical research; certainly the development of the science of medicine is justified. How much longer, however, should research efforts be directed towards discovering elusive 'specific etiologies,' the existence of which is becoming increasingly doubtful? Similarly, should we continue to direct research funding towards projects which assume that massed data can teach us how to deal with individuals? These are reductionist approaches, approaches which readily produce data because they simplify the human condition, but approaches which fail to make us healthier, happier people because of their neglect of so many of the factors which contribute to our state of health.

'For every disease' writes Lewis Thomas, 'there is a single mechanism which dominates all others. If one can find it, and then think one's way around it, one can control the disorder' (Thomas, 1979). Many billions of dollars have been spent for research studies which have attempted to uncover that 'single mechanism' which is thought to be primarily responsible for 'every' disease, while relatively few studies have been funded which have pursued answers to the phenomenon called illness by examining the multifactorial system which affects our state of health. The evolution of our current system for the delivery of health care services has also been guided by specific etiology doctrine, a doctrine which demands that illness be classified into specific diagnoses which require specific treatments without investigating the broader roots which contribute to the development of the state called illness.

According to Wildavsky, new 'administrative knowledge' can also transform American medicine. I suggest that the key to that knowledge lies not in the future, but in the past. 'Common practice' is not 'best practice' because modern physicians have lost the ecologic perspective. They treat diseases instead of people. They are silent until a disease develops; then they attempt to conquer the disease while ignoring the human needs of those whose bodies are diseased. Even worse, they ignore the human potential for self-healing. This potential, to be fully actualized, requires that a bond of trust be established between physician and patient, and that the patient becomes a full partner in a healing alliance.

Despite growing pressures for the return of Hippocrates' ecologic model, an institution which developed over the past century seals clinical medicine into a format inspired by the doctrine of specific etiology. That institution is medical specialism. We will examine the effects of specialization upon contemporary medical practice – effects which engender the necessity for Third Line Medicine to evolve into a major avenue of medical care – in Chapter Four.

CHAPTER 4
Specialism and its effects

> There are in truth no specialties in medicine
> since, to know many of the most important diseases,
> a man must be familiar with their manifestations
> in many organs.
>
> Sir William Osler
> 1849–1919

Physicians, in the Hippocratean model, are keen observers and scientists whose broad training and experience encompass all the many varieties of illness to which their patients are subject. Moreover they apply their knowledge with generosity and compassion. Physicians have not always lived up to the high standards the model espouses, any more than other professional groups have succeeded in maintaining the idealized standards of their respective models. Through the centuries, however, the model has been an inspiration for physicians and patients alike.

Fortunately, the high standards of the Hippocratean model were reinforced by the unique type of relationship established between physicians and their patients. These relationships were often the length of a lifetime, as many were established at the time of the patient's delivery and lasted until either of the two parties expired. Whole families were usually under one physician's care; in small towns, the entire town constituted one medical practice.

Physicians were highly visible in both their professional and personal lives as they played a central role in the community. For them, the boundary between professional and personal was blurred. When patients were seriously ill, they readily made house calls which brought them into the very center of family life. Neither were their personal lives ever entirely separated from the community, since they were available day or night, seven days a week, to handle emergencies.

With such great visibility, their dedication to their patients was obvious to the community. Patients got well, not only for themselves and their families, but also to gratify their doctors. The effective physician was the one who showed compassion as, until the past half century, physicians had little to offer in the way of effective medications.

While the general practitioner was, in many ways, the medical ecologist of the Hippocratean model, the modern specialist is more closely allied with specific etiology doctrine. George Rosen, author of *The Specialization of Medicine*, claims that specialization:.

> would hardly have taken place had not physicians accustomed themselves to the idea of distinct entities consisting of localized lesions connected with certain clinical pictures. . . . In short, the development and application of a concept of localized pathology laid the groundwork for modern specialism by providing a number of foci of interest in the field of medicine. (Rosen)

In other words, the move towards the development of medical specialties was instigated by the shift away from the ecologic model and towards the pathology-based model of the doctrine of specific etiology.

In addition to the shift away from the ecologic model, the trend towards specialism was necessitated by the tremendous explosion of scientific knowledge and the consequent development of medical technology which began to revolutionize medical care in the nineteenth century. As the armory of diagnostic and treatment procedures expanded, it soon became beyond the reach of the general practitioner; specialization was the inevitable result.

The publication of the Flexner report in 1910 did much to accelerate the trend towards specialization in the United States. Prior to World War One, the majority of American physicians entered general practice, while only a few major medical centers trained specialists. Even physicians who chose to study a medical specialty usually practiced general medicine for several years before embarking upon specialty training. This was in keeping with the older apprenticeship system of education which valued the senior general practitioners as they had seen the greatest variety of patients and had amassed the most clinical experience.

Flexner, by shifting the emphasis of medical education from learning by example to learning by the memorization of scientific techniques of evaluation and treatment, started the trend of replacing general practitioners in the teaching hospitals with the more scientific specialists. This raised the status of the specialists in the eyes of the students who began to aspire to more advanced medical training so that they could model themselves after their teachers. Further incentives to specialize came from the affluent sectors of the population which were more than willing to pay higher fees for receiving care from specialists.

Pressure built to develop a satisfactory means of distinguishing which physicians deserved to call themselves specialists. Accordingly, specialty boards were founded. Charged with developing certification procedures for their respective areas of expertise, the board assured that their diplomats would receive all the special professional and financial benefits which were starting to accrue to the practitioners of medical specialties.

By 1931, specialists had become a major force in American medicine, with 25 per cent of practicing physicians identifying themselves as practicing a medical specialty. World War Two further accelerated the trend towards specialization as board certified specialists were given higher rank, better assignments and additional pay. General physicians returning from military service sought specialty training in large numbers and residencies (hospital training programs in the medical specialties) expanded rapidly.

By the late 1940s, medical students had little or no contact with generalists throughout their medical training; specialists had replaced them as role models. Similarly, the teaching hospitals became exhibits of the latest in advanced medical technology. Patients were increasingly pre-screened so that students would be exposed primarily to those with rare and complex diseases, rather than to the common illnesses seen in general practice.

The customary period of general practice following basic

medical training lost favor as increasing numbers of medical graduates elected to begin specialty training immediately. The result was a still further decline in the numbers of general practitioners. In such a climate, the standing of GPs dropped precipitously until they were seen, in many circles, as 'drop-outs', certainly a far cry from the venerated country doctors of the past.

The trend towards specialization has yet to end. The American Medical Association agrees with the Association of American Medical Colleges that four years of medical training following college is no longer adequate to prepare the student for the independent practice of medicine (Levit *et al.*). In line with their position, virtually all United States medical school graduates today are undertaking specialty training and seeking specialty certification (ibid). At the present time, 70 per cent of all practicing American physicians identify themselves as medical specialists, and every four years the American Medical Association asks all practicing physicians to indicate which of eighty-five different specialties they consider to be their primary one.

Thus, in the United States, specialization has evolved from the exception to the norm. During the early years of specialty medicine, the system was relatively simple. First Line Medicine was provided by the general practitioners who referred their patients to specialists – the second line physicians – for those services which were beyond their grasp. (This remains the situation in England.)

Currently, as relatively few general practitioners remain, First Line Medicine in America is largely being provided by 'primary care' specialists such as family practitioners, internists and pediatricians. Second Line Medicine is also being practiced by these specialists along with specialists who limit themselves exclusively to second line patients (such as surgeons and oncologists). Patients requiring specialized services which their first line physician cannot provide are either referred to other specialists or, increasingly, seek them out directly.

In other words, the practice of American medicine has essentially become the practice of medical specialties. The trend towards ever-increasing specialization continues, however, with first line specialists either losing patients to second line subspecialists or becoming second line practitioners themselves.

One impetus for this trend is the belief of second line physicians that, because of their more specialized education, they are better equipped to deal with all aspects of patients' illnesses which fit into their specialty. Because of their feelings of superiority, they may even keep patients from returning to their first line physicians when their medical problems fall outside their personal specialties without realizing that this results in inferior, yet more expensive, medical care. One internist recently lamented this trend in a *Medical Economics* article:

> Many of my colleagues in primary care are concerned about the growing number of specialists who keep patients we've referred. . . . I'm concerned, too, and often angry – not just because it hits us in our pocketbooks, but because it disrupts a continuous relationship that's essential to good patient care. . . . Many . . . specialists don't appreciate primary care doctors. . . . They consider us simply triage officer to Their Majesties The Specialists. Because of that attitude, when the specialist doesn't keep the referring doctor's patient himself, he'll often send him along to a subspecialist colleague. . . . Most irksome, the patient is often directed to come back for checkups . . . to make sure [he] still doesn't have the disease [he] didn't have in the first place. (Paulshock)

Feelings of superiority are even causing second line physicians to squeeze their first line colleagues out of the hospitals. In a 1985 article, Harmon E. Holverson, a former president of the American Academy of Family Physicians, noted his concern that:

> . . . young family physicians are being denied hospital privileges in specialty areas where they have both documented training and experience. . . . What began about 10 years ago as an isolated incident here and there has metastasized into a nationwide pattern of discrimination . . . that threatens to stunt the careers of some 175 new FP's every year. . . . This disturbing turn of events harms more than the individual doctors involved. Patients

> suffer unnecessary discontinuity of care when specialists usurp the family doctors' places at bedside, and family medicine itself becomes a less appealing calling for young people every time an FP's wings are clipped. . . . Indeed, the number of residencies in the field . . . began declining two years ago. (Holverson)

Not knowing any better, patients have also been rushing to visit prestigious second line sub-specialists. Laments one internist:

> I could cite case after case in which my being a general internist just isn't good enough any more. Distrusting the internists' cognitive talent, educated laymen don't believe that clinical observation – no matter how skilled – is adequate for an accurate diagnosis. They want specialists in organs and diseases and expect a diagnosis via imaging techniques and tests, even if they're invasive. Forget the stethoscope – bring on the bronchoscope! (Wassersug)

Despite fears of a growing 'doctor glut' due to an increasing proportion of physicians in the American population, the number of physicians practicing First Line Medicine is actually declining. This trend towards ever-increasing specialization is so powerful that Karen Davis, chief planner at the US Department of Health, Education and Welfare, notes that the percentage of physicians entering second line medical practice is three times the percentage of patients requiring second line services. 'The system,' she says, 'is really out of whack.' (*New York Times* 30 July, 1978)

In 1976, the United States Congress, in an attempt to combat the trend away from First Line Medicine, passed legislation requiring American medical schools to provide an increasing proportion of first-year residency positions in the first line specialties. Even this legislation has been unsuccessful in reversing the trend, as a survey published in *The New England Journal of Medicine* reported that physicians who started training in first line specialties often switched to second line specialties later on (Wechsler *et al.*).

What is this continuing process of specialization doing to American medicine? There is no question that some form of specialization is necessary if the achievements of the research laboratory are to reach the public. The amount of study required to learn and to continually keep abreast of these achievements has long ago exceeded the ability of any one physician.

Unfortunately, the process of specialization which led to medical specialism as it exists in America today developed during the relatively brief era when physicians were mesmerized by the doctrine of specific etiology, and thus integral to it are all of the problems which are inherent in the doctrine. In fact, it is my contention that, despite its advantages, medical specialism has caused many, and perhaps most, of the ills suffered by modern medicine.

One result of such a process is that it is often a matter of luck as to whether a patient sees the proper specialists. Gene H. Stollerman, Professor of Medicine at Boston University, has written in a recent editorial that:

> Medical specialization has proliferated as fast as medical technology. It is not patients alone who are confused as to whom to consult and what to expect of their primary physician (if they are lucky enough to have one). Physicians vary greatly in their referral patterns, individually and as a group. For the primary physician, 'when to refer' is a constant issue. (Stollerman)

The lack of rational criteria for referrals is only one of many problems inherent in the current system of specialization. The increasingly heavy financial burden of the American consumer, for example, is in good measure a result of specialization. Specialists are wedded to high technology medicine, and the narrower the specialty, the more sophisticated and expensive the procedures. They must be familiar with, and accustomed to utilizing, the latest and most advanced diagnostic and therapeutic techniques if they are to maintain their reputations. Whenever the diagnosis is evasive or the illness is difficult to treat, specialists are tempted to use whatever tools are available to them within the bailiwick of their particular specialty before referring the patient away; thus the more tools which are developed, and the greater the number of second line specialties, the more expensive the cost of medical care.

However well versed they may be in their specialties, second line physicians are poorly prepared to evaluate diagnostic and therapeutic possibilities which are relatively non-specific. For example, some of the illnesses which involve multiple systems and are not infectious are more likely to escape their diagnostic nets than single-system illnesses. Similarly, the more natural remedies, since they are generally less specific in their effects than drugs and surgery, tend to be passed over in favor of the latter.

The more highly specialized they are, the less time that second line physicians have to devote to general medical education – but it is only their general medical education which enables them to maintain an ecologic perspective on their patients' illnesses. They concentrate instead upon reading the specific medical journals devoted to their specialty; journals whose editors are also likely to focus their personal reading upon that specialty. The same applies to their choice of medical conferences.

As a result, specialists see their patients in a distorted way, with the distortion depending upon the areas of emphasis and neglect in their medical education. With each specialty developing its own technical jargon as well as its own approach to diagnosis and treatment, different specialists can reach different conclusions about a patient's condition and select totally different treatments. Whether a patient with a complaint which is difficult to diagnose receives medication, exploratory surgery or psychotherapy often depends more upon the specialty of the practitioner than upon the ultimate merits of any particular treatment.

The specialist is not the only practitioner to suffer from a skewed perspective upon illness, for the development of a specialty affects, not only the practices of the new specialists, but also the practices of all other physicians. Robert A. Chase, a member of the National Board of Medical Examiners, notes that, when a new specialty develops,

> the non-specialists then begin to have doubts about their competence to deal with anything in that special area. Therefore, the non-specialist begins to refer all (both simple and complex) problems within that special area to

> the certified superspecialist. This in fact has a tendency to diminish the non-specialist's own competence by lack of exposure and experience so that he subsequently must refer all such cases to the specialist. (Chase)

Specialization, therefore, not only produces physicians with narrow areas of knowledge and expertise, but also narrows the area of competence and expertise of the remaining generalists – as well as the area of competence and expertise of all other specialists whose areas of specialization touch upon the area of the new specialist. How deleterious this is depends upon the manner of specialization more than upon the development of specialization itself.

Least deleterious has been the restriction of medical practice to a single life stage. Pediatrics has been the major example of such a restriction, although geriatrics and adolescent medicine are other examples which have recently been gaining in popularity. This type of specialization suffers from the loss of continuity through the life cycle. Children lose what has been their life-long relationship with their pediatrician in the middle of adolescent turbulence to have to start a new physician-patient relationship. Such a change weakens the traditional bond between physician and patient and may add to the natural instability of this life stage for certain vulnerable youngsters. Otherwise, this type of practice restriction retains the broad viewpoint of ecologic medicine.

A second type of specialization is the restriction of medical practice to limited forms of treatment. Surgery and nuclear medicine are examples of this type of restriction. Physicians who practice only one type of treatment often have brief, limited and relatively impersonal relationships with their patients since their relationship with them terminates at the completion of their course of treatment. In addition, their predominant concern is in determining whether their treatment is appropriate for the patient and, if so, in performing the treatment skillfully. For this type of specialist, causative factors are considered irrelevant and are thus neglected even though those factors are continuing to influence the course of the patient's illness during their term of care.

The third type of specialization restricts the specialist to a single organ system or portion of the body. Cardiologists and vascular surgeons typify this type which embodies some of the distortions noted for the first and second types. It also adds another serious distortion. These specialists figuratively dissect their patients into parts as if those parts were capable of a separate existence. This distortion compromises their ability to appreciate the full impact of the multiple physical and psychological influences upon those parts from the rest of the body as well as from the external environment. Insofar as they cannot appreciate these influences, they also cannot attempt to manipulate them to foster the process of healing.

The last type of specialization restricts the specialist to dealing with 'mental illnesses'. The distortion created by this type of specialization, which is the basis for the specialty of psychiatry, lies in the premise that disturbances in mental processes and behavior are sufficiently distinct from disturbances in bodily processes to warrant specialized assessment and treatment. The *raison d'être* of psychiatry, therefore, is based on the Cartesian separation of mind from body.

Mental illnesses are currently defined as illnesses 'with psychologic or behavioral manifestations and/or impairment in functioning due to a social, psychologic, genetic, physical/chemical or biological disturbance.' (*A Psychiatric Glossary*) In actual practice, psychiatrists deal primarily with people who complain of emotional distress or who exhibit abnormal behaviors.

Uncertain of its identity, psychiatry has been caught between its fascination with mental mechanisms and its medical roots (Fink). Since theoretical mental processes are too ethereal to be studied with the instruments of hard science, its ties to psychodynamics (the study of mental forces in action) have, in this age of science, relegated it to a step-child position in the medical family.

Sir Isaac Newton once lamented that, 'I can calculate the matters of heavenly bodies, but not the madness of people.' Sigmund Freud, the father of psychiatry, was equally at a loss to validate his observations with acceptable scientific studies. According to Murray Bowen, Clinical Professor of Psychiatry at Georgetown University,

> Freud tried to make his observations fit a medical model, but he ran into subject matter that he couldn't measure. . . . Scientists didn't buy it. They think that if you can't measure something, you can't know it. Most medical scientists consider psychiatry mumbo jumbo. (ibid.)

Even today, psychiatry has yet to develop a theory which meets the criteria of scientific theories in the physical sciences – namely a description of relationships or behaviors that are repeatable and predictable. In fact, despite its advocacy by numerous psychiatrists and their patients, the hypothesis that psychodynamic psychotherapy is effective in the treatment of mental illness has yet to receive definitive scientific validation (Parloff).

Contemporary physicians, raised on a diet of specific etiology doctrine, cite this failure as justification for their anti-psychological orientation. They believe that whatever their validating instruments have failed to prove valid is invalid until proven otherwise. Poorly regarded by the rest of the medical community, psychiatry is gradually dwindling in influence as fewer and fewer medical students choose psychiatric residencies (Nielsen). In the words of the *American Medical Association News*, 'there seems to be an almost general bias against psychiatry.' (Stacey)

Whatever respect psychiatry has developed within the medical community, it has developed, not because of its interest in mental processes, but because of its long-standing ties to neurology. Investigation of the mind as a manifestation of a functioning brain and utilization of biologically based treatments such as pharmacotherapy and electroconvulsive ('shock') therapy are approaches which can be studied with the same investigative tools as are employed in the other medical specialties and have permitted psychiatry to retain its fraternity membership. In addition, by emphasizing its biological roots, it has been able to distinguish itself from its sister field of psychology (which avidly competes with it for patients).

Thus psychiatry has been tempted, and sometimes succumbs to the temptation, to orient itself towards biology. Yet psychiatrists sense that there is an inherent danger in assuming that orientation. As we look back, whenever a specific biological treatment was identified for a sub-group of patients with psychosis, those patients were re-labeled and swallowed up by other medical specialties. Examples are the psychoses which are now known to be due to endocrine disorders and vitamin deficiencies. In addition, non-psychiatric physicians utilize the same drugs for emotional disorders as do psychiatrists. Thus, while non-medical mental health professionals increasingly nibble away at psychiatry's territorial claims regarding psychological treatments, non-psychiatric physicians are nibbling away at its claims regarding biological treatments.

Perhaps because of such threats to its survival, psychiatry has restricted its interest in the mind-body interface to certain limited areas which are at once too medical for non-medical mental health professionals and too psychological for non-psychiatric physicians. In psychiatric practice, interest in psychological influences upon disease processes has been largely restricted to a small and arbitrary group of 'psychosomatic disorders'. In the chapters to come, we shall review some of the increasingly massive evidence that there are, in fact, relatively few illnesses in which the psyche plays no role in their genesis, and fewer still in which the psyche plays no role in their clinical course. Yet the co-editor of the authoritative *Comprehensive Textbook of Psychiatry* has recently written that: 'Representatives from both fields of study, psyche and soma, have agreed for more than 100 years that, in a small body of disorders, emotional and somatic activities overlap.' (Kaplan)

Despite their narrow view of psychological influences upon disease, psychiatrists have demonstrated increasing interest in the emerging specialty of liaison psychiatry. Liaison psychiatrists assist in the care of patients with physical illnesses and often work on the medical, rather than on the psychiatric, hospital wards. As psychiatrists, they are concerned with the psychological aspects of illness and are usually called in when the patient's physicians become aware of significant psychological issues. They deal with a variety of clinical problems: patients who have difficulty in coping with their illnesses, physicians who have difficulty in coping with their patients, and patients whose emotional states have an obvious bearing on the course of their illnesses (Lipowski).

Liaison psychiatry is one of the few areas in which

psychiatrists are fairly well protected from infringement by other professionals. As physicians, they have more tools for dealing with medical patients in hospital settings than their non-medical colleagues. At the same time, their willingness to spend time with emotionally needy patients is welcomed by other physicians who wish to be rescued of that responsibility and who have had little training to prepare them to assume it.

Psychiatric treatment thus bridges the mind-body split through the development of three sub-specialties. In biological psychiatry, somatic treatments are utilized for psychological problems. In psychosomatic medicine, treatment is directed at the 'small body' of disorders in which the mind is believed to have affected either the actual functional state of the body or merely the patients' perceptions of that state while, in liaison psychiatry, treatment is directed at the medical patient with emotional or behavioral problems.

The positive contributions of these three sub-specialties are undeniable. Unfortunately, the development of a single specialty concerned with 'mental illness' has removed the responsibility for dealing with the complex mental aspects of *all* illness from non-psychiatric physicians without transferring but a small portion of that responsibility, as encompassed in the three sub-specialties I have described, to the territory of psychiatry.

Modern physicians, concerned with deciding whether a patient has either a mental or a physical illness, often neglect to deal with psychological issues which have not produced abnormal behavior or inappropriate emotional states. They forget that the psyche has a powerful influence upon the course of any illness, an influence which may be as powerful as any specific treatment they may prescribe. They forget that the quality of their relationships with their patients is central to strengthening psychic healing influences, and fail to attempt to develop a trusting, caring, collaborative relationship with them.

The social and psychological aspects of illness are so commonly neglected, not because they have been proven to be irrelevant, but because they fail to lend themselves to the reductionist approach characteristic of the scientific study of physical phenomena and advocated by specific etiology doctrine. Bias against dealing with these important aspects of illness shows up clearly in the manner in which physicians are paid for their time, since time spent with patients is rewarded far less than time spent on impersonal procedures. A urologist, for example, earns *ten times* as much money while operating as for an office visit. According to an article in *The New England Journal of Medicine*,

> time spent in office visits – time for listening, observing, deciding, advising, explaining, counseling and instructing – is in fact the least highly rewarded activity in fee schedules. . . . Present fee schedules offer physicians excessively strong incentives to furnish technical services and insufficient encouragement to perform as the patient's advisor, counselor, and health advocate. (Almy)

Walter Cannon, the great physiologist, warned physicians half a century ago against dichotomizing disease into those problems with known pathophysiology and those that leave no distinct anatomic alterations (Cannon). Today, however, specific etiology doctrine dictates that physical health is separate from mental health, with the former given far more importance than the latter. Medical insurance plans not only encourage surgery and highly technologic procedures by readily disbursing large sums of money, but visits with psychiatrists are determined to be worth far less per hour than visits with most other specialists – and are often entirely excluded from otherwise comprehensive policies.

Even when insurance coverage for psychological problems is available, the insurance industry refuses to reimburse patients for the cost of psychiatric services unless their psychiatrists diagnose them as suffering from a mental illness. This places both the doctor and the patient on the horns of a dilemma. If the doctor decides that the patient is 'mentally ill', there is insurance coverage, but the patient will have to live with the stigma of that label. On the other hand, if the doctor decides that the patient could benefit from treatment, but is not 'mentally ill', the insurance company may refuse to pay for services.

Thus, when patients are accepted for psychiatric care, they are usually labeled as mentally ill, even in instances when that designation is unwarranted. This practice is consistent with the doctrine of specific etiology since, according to the doctrine, physicians deal only with illness; all illness is caused by disease, and all disease is either physical or mental.

Because psychiatrists are often derided or not affordable, and non-psychiatric physicians are discouraged from spending time talking, patients with emotional problems are encouraged to redefine their problems in physical terms. An insurance policy, for example, may not cover the treatment of anxiety, but it will cover the treatment of the physical manifestations of anxiety such as palpitations, nausea and dizziness.

This unfortunate pressure on patients to define emotionally-based symptoms in somatic terms has had a major effect upon primary care by causing overutilization of first line physicians. In an English study, over 50 per cent of patients with psychiatric problems were found to present initially with physical complaints (Koiton). Their physicians may fail to evaluate the psychosocial stress which underlies their complaints and may reinforce the problem by arranging unnecessary laboratory tests, clinic visits, hospitalizations and even surgery (ibid.). Studies have found that between 9 per cent and 37 per cent of patients presenting to first line physicians have significant psychopathology which was missed by them (Cooper and Sylph, Brown and Fry).

Another possibility is that these patients may seek out or be referred to second line physicians. Palpitations may be evaluated by a cardiologist, nausea by a gastroenterologist, and dizziness either by a neurologist or an otolaryngologist or both. These specialists need to complete work-ups which are both extensive and expensive so as to protect themselves from the possibility of malpractice suits. Then, since they are ill-prepared to teach anxious patients how to master their anxieties, they will probably treat them with tranquilizers and send them on their way.

Evidence for the deleterious effects of encouraging patients to define their illnesses in physical terms comes from studies investigating the effects of adding psychiatric services to medical facilities. Their conclusion: the provision of psychiatric services actually results in a net *reduction* in the cost of providing medical care! This finding appears to be due to the dramatic decrease in the utilization of medical services once psychiatric services are introduced (Jones and Vischi, Schlesinger *et al.*).

Patients with obvious psychopathology have a different problem. Instead of the avoidance of psychiatric consultation which otherwise occurs, these patients may not even have adequate medical evaluations before being rushed to psychiatrists. One author, for example, has demonstrated that between one-third and one-half of all physicians referring patients to psychiatrists act as if the psychiatrists were first line physicians, often neglecting to take histories or give their patients physical examinations before sending their patients on to them (Johnson). Another has reviewed a dozen studies and concluded that 50 per cent of referring physicians had not diagnosed their patients' physical illnesses before initiating a psychiatric referral (Koranyi).

Psychiatrists are no more likely to do a comprehensive evaluation of the relationship between psychological and somatic factors than their colleagues. Emotional symptoms are likely to be viewed as psychogenic. Even when a medical evaluation has not been performed by first line physicians, psychiatrists may neglect to perform one. One study found that less than 35 per cent of practicing psychiatrists physically examine their patients; in fact, 32 per cent of the psychiatrists surveyed indicated that they did not feel competent to perform a physical examination (McIntyre and Romano).

Richard C. W. Hall of the Medical College of Wisconsin notes that:

> Many [psychiatric] residents complete their training without being systematically instructed in a detailed fashion in the procedures necessary to accomplish adequate initial medical evaluation of their patients. The current mode of outpatient psychiatric practice in this country, in general, accepts the absence of underlying medical illness as a cause for psychiatric symptoms. (*APA Psychiatric News* 6 February 1981)

The tragic result is that significant numbers of psychiatric patients have a mental illness which is due to, or exacerbated by, unrecognized physical illness. Among psychiatric outpatients, Hall and his colleagues have found that over 9 per cent have psychiatric symptoms caused by previously unrecognized illnesses (Hall *et al.*, 1978). This means that almost one out of ten patients now seeing psychiatrists in their offices are receiving inappropriate treatment! The statistics for psychiatric in-patients, most of whom come from the lower socio-economic class, are even more striking. Hall and his colleagues have reported that, for this population, almost *one-half* (46 per cent) were thought to have medical illnesses that directly caused or greatly exacerbated their symptoms and were consequently responsible for their admission. In addition, another one-third (34 per cent) were found to be suffering from a medical illness requiring treatment which had been missed until the time of the study (Hall *et al.* 1980).

The sad fact is that the process of specialization is continuing to ravage the ecologic model. The greater the degree of specialization, the less the model can be appreciated. We are losing what Hippocrates considered to be one of the physician's most valuable assets: comprehension of the total ecosystem which surrounds and influences the course of all illness. According to the authors of *A Short History of Medicine*:

> It is not merely the enormous bulk of writings on science and medicine that forms the main deterrent to the general comprehension of its principles. Probably since at least the eighteenth century the mass of scientific detail has been beyond the grasp of any one mind. . . . In approaching our own age we have found increasing difficulty in discussing rational medicine as a single channel of thought. It spreads into a delta which tends to diverge ever wider, though still the many mouths may inosculate. This diffusion, brought about by increasing specialization, cannot go on indefinitely without defeating the objects for which specialism arose. (Singer and Underwood)

Specialism is the glue which cements modern medicine into specific etiology doctrine. It is fundamental to our system of practice and serves a most important purpose – that of making the latest and most sophisticated level of medical expertise available to the public. Its deficits, however, are serious ones, and the development of new specialties, far from correcting the deficits, only compounds them further.

As is the case with specialization, methods of practicing medicine are less based upon medical science than upon the nature of the prevailing institutions – institutions whose deficits can be traced to the pernicious influence of the doctrine of specific etiology. The actual role of science in the practice of medicine will be the subject of our next chapter.

CHAPTER 5
Science and the medical model

> The secret of the care of the patient
> is in caring for the patient.
>
> FRANCIS WELD PEABODY
> 1881–1927

We live in the age of science. The applications of scientific research permeate every aspect of our existence, from our transports to our foods, from our means of communication to our weaponry. Basic sciences are taught in our elementary schools, while the media deluge us with titillating glimpses of the newest and the latest in scientific advances. Throughout the world, the assumption prevails that scientific advances will better the lives of all of us; thus an investment in scientific research is believed to be an investment for our future.

What is science? The word is derived from the Latin word *scientia* (*sciens*, the present participle of *scire*, 'to know'.) Authorities seem to argue that science can be defined as *an objective, logical and systematic method of analysis of phenomena, devised to permit the accumulation of reliable knowledge.* (Lastrucci) A method rather than a philosophy, it is not committed to any theory or philosophical position. Neither does it discover 'truth' in any absolute or ultimate sense; rather it tests hypotheses to determine the extent of their validity. It has no lasting allegiance to its own conclusions for, as soon as the results of new experiments question old conclusions, it changes its position to remain consistent with the accumulated evidence.

Conversion of the emphasis in training medical practitioners from the transfer and personal development of empirical knowledge to the mastery of scientific literature has had profound implications upon patient care. We have benefited greatly from the increased emphasis on science for, without science, we tend to delude ourselves. We mistake coincidence for causation. We choose complexity when simplicity is superior. We harm when we believe we are helping. Our biases distort our vision and we continue to reinvent the wheel.

It is not the fault of science, but of the manner in which many modern practitioners of medicine misuse science which, I submit, is responsible for many of medicine's current failings. Science is merely a method of validating hypotheses, a way of proceeding on a quest for knowledge. It is a slow, ponderous means of investigation which is incapable of dealing directly with the complexities of the living organism. Instead, in order to be able to investigate its subject, it must select only aspects of the organism's characteristics in the hope that, once enough aspects of the organism are understood, the nature of the organism itself will be comprehended (ibid.). Forgotten is the fact that the characteristics of an organism which has been torn apart into simple units may bear little resemblance to those of the functioning whole.

Science, thus, demands simplification; yet it does not specify which characteristics of an object should be selected for study. Until the hypothetical time when the object is entirely understood, the content of science depends upon the choice of questions which are asked and hypotheses which are formulated for testing. These decisions are made outside the realm of science; they are based on the personal beliefs, values and priorities of the scientist. The situation is much like the parable of the blind man and the elephant. Each man examines a different part of the animal as each stands in a different location. Since they are unable to comprehend the nature of the complete animal, each man reaches a different conclusion concerning the nature of the elephant based on the characteristic he has examined.

The prevalent view is that the application of science protects us from our biases. The truth is that scientific research is commonly utilized as a means of fostering or discrediting particular orientations or value systems. This point has been made most cogently by Thomas Kuhn who, in *The Structure of Scientific Revolutions*, traced the character and success of science to the social organization and social psychology of scientists. 'Whatever scientific progress may be,' he writes, 'we must account for it by examining the nature of the scientific *group*, discovering what it values, what it tolerates, and what it disdains.' (Kuhn)

Increased reliance upon scientific investigation as the basis for claims of clinical efficacy has failed to eradicate the effects of personal bias upon medical judgment. Studies demonstrating the superiority of treatment A over treatment B, for example, may only mean that those in favor of treatment A have been more successful in designing studies which demonstrate the superiority of their favorite treatment – perhaps because they have greater financial resources than those in favor of treatment B. Reviewers can hardly present a balanced review when studies by those favoring treatment B are lacking; besides, what assurance is there that their reviews are unbiased?

There are five levels of information which are available to physicians to aid in making clinical decisions. None of these levels, unfortunately, fully protects them or their patients from the danger of being influenced by biased conclusions.

Level one consists of *anecdotal reports* which suggest hypotheses. Johnny has an illness which disappears after he is given some untested remedy. Did the remedy cure him? Many people might believe that it did. On the other hand, there are other explanations for Johnny's improvement. The disease may have been self-limiting, so that Johnny would have become well even if he didn't receive the remedy. Johnny's illness may have responded to the 'kindness' of his physician, or Johnny may have been doing something else at the same time as he took the remedy which caused his illness to remit. There may even be adverse effects from the remedy in certain people which are unrecognized but which Johnny was fortunate to have avoided. Thus the mere coincidence of timing between introduction of the treatment and healing can do little more than suggest that the treatment may be of value.

Data which are considered to be more scientific can be gleaned from level two studies, which consist of *retrospective data analyses*. These are a form of scientific research which examines data which have already been accumulated to discover differences between groups which may explain different treatment outcomes. These studies have a major advantage over anecdotal reports, since they permit the use of the power of statistical analyses to discover, for example, whether the observed differences between groups are significant, i.e. unlikely to be due to chance. However, even though level two studies are often widely accepted because of their use of statistical methodology, they are still fraught with possibilities for incorrect conclusions (Feinstein *et al.*).

Level three consists of scientific *experiments*. At the present time, the most popular, highly respected type of experiment is the randomized, double-blind controlled study which randomly divides patients into two groups. One of these groups, the experimental group, receives the treatment being investigated; the other, the control group, receives either a standard treatment or a placebo (a 'dummy' treatment), and the results of treatment in the two groups are compared. Since neither the researchers nor the patients are told who is in which group, personal biases are thought to be eliminated from the results.

Such a conclusion is terribly naive. The double-blind controlled study is indeed a considerable advance over lower levels of information – but it suffers from serious flaws. For example, many valuable treatments cannot be investigated in this manner because it is impossible to create a placebo treatment which appears to patients to be the same as the experimental treatment. Examples are studies of DMSO (which produces a characteristic taste and body odor) and studies of psychotherapy, treatments which have been unfairly disparaged by many physicians who refuse to approve of any procedure which has not been validated by this form of research study.

Even for treatments which are appropriate for double-blind studies, there is considerable evidence that both patients and researchers can often figure out who is in which group – although researchers rarely bother to find out if this has occurred (Brownell and Stunkard, Byington *et al.*). Since, whenever this happens, the results of the study become meaningless because placebo effects cannot be separated out, the conclusions suggested by many of the studies published in the literature are actually invalid.

Yet another deficit of the double-blind study is its assumption that the placebo effect is a unitary phenomenon. The truth is that the effect of a placebo is not standardized, but depends upon a number of factors which are specific to each investigation, such as the interaction between the personality of the patient and the treatment milieu (Shipman *et al.*).

Thus, unless it can be shown that the placebo effect in two studies was identical, those studies cannot be compared. In fact, the demonstration that an experimental treatment was better than the placebo is only relevant in similar situations with similar patients – and therefore fails to provide definitive proof that that treatment will be any better than a placebo for a particular patient in a clinical setting.

Because only certain kinds of phenomena can be studied by double-blind studies, and because the results of published double-blind studies may be misleading, such studies can be no more than aids, when they are available, in helping physicians to make therapeutic decisions. Unfortunately, they tend to be worshipped by specific etiologists because they appear to offer simple conclusions about what they consider to be simple issues.

Information level four is characterized by *reviews of published studies*. It is generally accepted that research findings are considered to be preliminary until they are confirmed by other laboratories. As similar studies mount, reviewers critically assess the accumulating evidence and draw conclusions. In contrast to the precautions against bias taken in level three studies, level four reviews are unprotected from the biases of the reviewer and journal editors; thus different reviewers can reach different conclusions by examining the same group of studies. In practice, the reviews published by the most prestigious reviewers in the most prestigious journals are those which become generally accepted.

Over the passage of time, the most widely accepted conclusions from level four reviews become reflected in the information published in textbooks. *Textbooks*, therefore, represent level five, the highest, most respected, level of information. Like level four reviews, they are subject to the biases of the writer.

The higher the level of information, the longer the delay between the time that new information is discovered and the time that it is disseminated. This delay is due to the time needed for validation and may easily take a decade or longer between levels one and five. In addition, the higher the information level, the less controversial that information is considered to be. All would agree that physicians should feel free to utilize data from level five in their practices. In fact, it is considered to be the responsibility of physicians to be aware of all relevant level five information.

All would also agree that the best physicians keep abreast of information appearing at levels two to four. The lower the level, the more controversial it is for them to utilize that data in their practices. Most controversial is the utilization of information from level one (anecdotal reports), and physicians are generally discouraged from its application.

In the simplistic medical model championed by the specific etiologists, the practice of medicine is merely the application of medical science to the treatment of disease. Anything else is quackery. The truth is that medical science, as valuable as it is, is grossly inadequate to the task of providing a single foundation for medical practice, and additional sources of guidance are imperative. Even if we examine the decisions made by typical physicians in practice, their basis in science is a flimsy one, for a recent report commissioned by the United States Congress concluded that only 10 to 20 per cent of such decisions are based on the results of scientific investigations (Office of Technology Assessment, US Congress)!

Half a century ago, Sir William Osler asserted that:

> The practice of medicine is an art, based on science. Working with science, for science, it has not reached, perhaps never will, the dignity of a complete science, with exact laws, like astronomy or engineering. Is there no science of medicine? Yes, but in parts only, such as anatomy and physiology. (Osler)

Since science can only assist physicians in their task of reaching diagnostic and therapeutic decisions, the model of illness upon which physicians base these decisions will be very influential. Today, with the doctrine of specific etiology serving as the basis for the medical model, medical education consists of two years of study of the most scientific parts of medicine followed by two years of study with a succession of medical specialists, with each specialist viewing the patient through the narrow lens of his or her specialty. Medical students spend little time learning the sophistication of their art; the personal aspects of illness are studied primarily in terms of separating the 'hysterics' from the patients with 'real' diseases.

By the time that physicians have graduated from medical school, they have acquired a mass of scientific knowledge but remain naive about the non-scientific aspects of medical practice. They have little understanding of how their diagnostic and treatment decisions may be influenced by economic factors, value systems, or the quality of their physician-patient relationships. They may even be ill-equipped to decide for themselves the scientific merits of new procedures, since they have been trained to accept the viewpoints of their professors and may not have received adequate training in the methods of properly evaluating scientific studies.

Textbook medicine has become the standard of practice for contemporary physicians. Instead of seeking to understand *why* their patients became ill, they seek to classify them according to textbook descriptions of diseases. They are too uncomfortable with dealing with the patients in human terms; instead they seek impersonal means of treating them. They fail to recognize their over-reliance on surgery, technology and pharmacology, and counter their patients' alienation by further distancing themselves.

Fortunately, despite the stranglehold which specific etiology doctrine has had upon the practice of medicine, this past decade has witnessed a gradual revival of ecologic concepts and practices. Science has provided the impetus for the revival – just as science had provided the impetus for the development of a medical model based upon the doctrine of specific etiology a century ago. It is ironic that, since the doctrine of specific etiology was hailed as the model which introduced science into modern medicine, modern medical scientists no longer even consider the doctrine to be consistent with scientific principles, principles which have undergone a major revolution since Descartes. In fact, contemporary scientific models bear a surprisingly close resemblance to the ecologic model. Half a century ago, Morris R. Cohen and Ernest Nagel warned of two common violations of modern scientific principles. The first is the *fallacy of pseudo simplicity*:

> It is supposed that because a given theory expresses any important truth about a subject, every other theory must be false. If social institutions and customs are a function of the prevailing means of production, it does not follow that these have not geographical, psychological, or political determinants as well. (Cohen and Nagel)

The reductionist viewpoint of specific etiology doctrine suffers from this fallacy. For example, the doctrine was modeled on the germ theory of disease which provided the basis for immunization and the development of antibiotics – treatments which, proponents claim, were responsible for the dramatic decline in the prevalence of fatal infections. We now have evidence, however, that most of the common infections (tuberculosis, pneumonia, scarlet fever, measles, pertussis, etc.) had declined in incidence to a low level even before these specific treatments were introduced. The major factors responsible for the improvement of health during the past three centuries, according to Thomas McKeown, Professor of Social Medicine Emeritus at the University of Birmingham in England, were 'the provision of food, protection from hazards, and limitation of numbers.' (McKeown) Multiple *non-specific* factors, therefore, had fostered the transmission of infections. Once all the etiological factors are appreciated, the role of the specific pathologic agent dwindles in importance.

This same fallacy of pseudo simplicity has prevented specific etiologists from dealing effectively with the new killer diseases. Tuberculosis, pneumonia and influenza, the major causes of death from disease in the past, now cause less than 2 per cent of the health problem they caused in 1900 (Fries). As the incidence of fatal infections has declined, a new group of diseases, which had previously been less common, arose to replace them as major causes of death from disease. These are the degenerative diseases, the most common of which are arteriosclerotic heart disease, cancer and diabetes mellitus. Since, in contrast to the infectious diseases, these diseases do not require a specific pathologic agent to be present for their initiation or progression, the specific etiologists have found them to be vastly more difficult to understand. Rather than admit that these diseases may result from the interplay of multiple etiologic factors, many of which have been clearly identified, they persist in searching for the elusive 'fundamental' cause which they expect to be specific for each disease.

While the doctrine of specific etiology has promulgated this fallacy in the field of medicine, medical research has repeatedly confirmed a multi-factorial, systems model as the one best able to explain the genesis of illness. For example, through selective breeding techniques, a strain of mice has been produced which is genetically predisposed to breast cancer. Investigators have been able to achieve drastic variations in the incidence of breast cancer in these mice by manipulating any of a number of factors:

1 Virus: Exposure to a virus in the mother's breast milk is required for tumor development.
2 Hormones: Females only develop the tumor after the stress of repeated breeding and lactation. Males develop the tumor if injected with estrogenic (female) hormones.
3 Nutrition: Tumor incidence is drastically reduced by placing the mice on a low calorie diet (Dubos).

Specific etiology doctrine would identify the 'milk virus' as the factor responsible for the genesis of the cancer. Indeed, if we could prevent the transmission of the virus, or if we could develop an effective anti-viral vaccine, the cancer could be prevented. If, however, these treatment alternatives are unavailable, knowledge of the other etiologic factors (genetic predisposition, sex hormones and nutrition) gives us additional measures by which the disease can be prevented.

The other violation, according to Cohen and Nagel, is the *fallacy of reduction*. Science does not simply reduce objects into their constituent elements, but: 'analyzes objects into elements that are related to each other in certain ways, so that if the elements were related in different ways, they would constitute *other* objects.' (Cohen and Nagel)

Similarly, Einstein and Infeld have noted that, in nineteenth-century physics, scientists endeavored 'to describe all natural phenomena in terms of simple forces between unalterable objects (Einstein and Infeld). Twentieth century physics, on the other hand, recognizes that it is not the behavior of bodies, but the behavior of something between them, that is the *field*, which is essential for ordering and understanding events.

Fritjof Capra, a theoretical physicist at the Lawrence Berkeley Laboratory of the University of California, writes that:

> The material world appears not as Newton saw it, but as a harmonious 'organic' whole, whose parts are only defined through their interrelations. The universe of the modern physicist, like that of the eastern mystic, is engaged in a continuous cosmic dance; it is a system of inseparable, ever-moving parts, of which the observer is an integral part. (Capra)

Thus, in modern physics, scientists are no longer merely spectators but are active participants in the system they are studying. Observers in different systems moving in respect to each other will perceive the world differently; yet they are each involved in establishing physical reality.

The new philosophy of science is that *all* observations are made in the light of theoretical preconceptions. The subjective, personal data derived from informal observation, long stigmatized by specific etiologists, are now returning to respectability as legitimate methods of obtaining scientific knowledge in areas (such as the behavioral sciences) where much of the phenomena cannot be reduced to the format required for the type of study requiring the isolation of only a few variables (Hine *et al.*). Psychosocial factors are no longer seen by the new scientists as embarrassing constructs which will be abandoned once they can be explained in the language of the physical sciences. Their claim is that subjecting the social sciences to scientific standards developed for the physical sciences is inappropriate. According to a recent article in *The American Journal of Psychiatry*:

> In the natural sciences, precise, quantitative research is successful in developing knowledge of many simple, lawful, and predictive relationships between phenomena. In contrast, most psychosocial events cannot be usefully studied in the same way as the activities of subatomic particles.... Although the foregoing phenomena are

> incredibly complex . . , the complexity of the events involved in psychotherapy is so much greater that a qualitative change is required in our concepts of research methods and criteria of acceptable knowledge. A more inclusive and relaxed conception of 'science' is needed. (ibid)

Specific etiologists fail to realize that subjecting the human sciences to the same tests as the natural sciences is much like rating apples on a scale developed for oranges. Their essence is lost when we demand specification in precise, quantitative terms – for much of their essence is found in the world of the subjective, in the world of qualitative differences, in the world of terms such as God, love and hope which can only be defined by consensus. One author has even gone so far as to suggest that the imitation of the methods, language and standards of the physical sciences by the social sciences is not true science, but 'scientism.' (Hayek)

The new scientists, strongly commited to a systems approach, view psychosocial issues as one level of analysis which is as legitimate as any other level of analysis. Harold J. Morowitz, Professor of Molecular Biophysics and Biochemistry at Yale University, believes that the time has come to integrate the perspectives of psychology, biology and physics. He sees such an integration as a great epistemological circle which starts and ends with the mind:

> First, the human mind, including consciousness and reflective thought, can be explained by activities of the central nervous system, which, in turn, can be reduced to the biological structure and function of that physiological system. Second, biological phenomena at all levels can be totally understood in terms of atomic physics, that is, through the action and interaction of the component atoms of carbon, nitrogen, oxygen, and so forth. Third, and last, atomic physics, which is now understood most fully by means of quantum mechanics, must be formulated with the mind as a primitive component of the system. (Morowitz)

In the reductionist approach of specific etiology doctrine, research studies commonly investigate processes shared by groups and view individual variances as irrelevant. In the systems approach of the new scientists, individuality is given as much relevance as are the processes shared by groups. While medical research neglected individuality in the nineteenth century, awareness of its importance was shared by enlightened individuals. One of these was John Abercrombie, First Physician to His Majesty in Scotland who, back in 1834, lamented that:

> There is great difficulty in medicine tracing effects to their true causes, and causes to their true effects. The same cause may appear to produce in different instances different diseases, or no diseases at all; and . . . a disease may seem to subside under the use of a remedy which, in a similar case, fails to produce the smallest benefit. (Abercrombie)

Leo Tolstoy, the great Russian novelist, warned against textbook medicine in *War and Peace*:

> No single disease can be fully understood in a living person; for every living person has his individual peculiarities and always his own peculiar, new, complex complaints unknown to medicine – not a disease of the lungs, of the kidneys, of the skin, of the heart, and so on, as described in medical books, but a disease that consists of one out of the innumerable combinations of ailments of those organs.

Even Louis Pasteur, whose germ theory of infection was to serve as the prototype of the doctrine of specific etiology, was opposed to the tenets of the doctrine. According to Pasteur, the disease could not be understood without knowledge of the individual who became infected, since not only the organism, but also the host's susceptibility to infection would determine whether an infection would develop. He believed that the body's biochemical and physiological state, and even the person's emotional attitudes, profoundly affected the course and outcome of all infectious diseases.

Unfortunately, there continues to be relatively little scientific exploration into the personal aspects of disease from a biological perspective. An exception has been the work of

Roger J. Williams whose major contributions to nutritional science have earned him worldwide recognition. Williams notes that, 'if medicine were a pure science it would perhaps be interested in hypothetical average people. Being an applied science, its interest must be in real people who are of many sorts and suffer from many sorts of disease.' (Williams, 1975)

It has become time to abandon the narrow, disease-orientation promulgated by the doctrine of specific etiology and to return to the concept of healing the ill. Prince Charles, in addressing the British Medical Association (December, 1982) has noted that:

> By concentrating on smaller and smaller fragments of the body, modern medicine perhaps loses sight of the patient as a whole human being, and by reducing health to the mechanical functioning it is no longer able to deal with the phenomenon of healing. . . . The term 'healer' is viewed with suspicion and the concepts of health and healing are probably not generally discussed enough in medical schools. But to reincorporate the notion of healing into the practice of medicine does not necessarily mean that medical science will have to be less scientific. Through the centuries healing has been practised by folk-healers who are guided by traditional wisdom that sees illness as a disorder of the whole person, involving not only the patient's body, but his mind, his self-image, his dependence on the physical environment, as well as his relation to the cosmos. . . .

The more we look at the total situation, the more complex the patient's situation appears. Science has helped to clarify this picture, but it provides medical practitioners with only pieces of knowledge which, taken naively, lead to distortions in their appreciation of the nature of illness as well as the means of best moving their patients back towards health. These distortions are not the fault of science, but the fault of those who misuse science in the mistaken belief that medical practice must be based solely upon science.

The problem is one of the tail wagging the dog. Science should not be worshipped as the source of all knowledge; rather it should be incorporated into the art of healing. For all of its brilliance in uncovering truth, science will never replace intuition, communication, hope or compassion. 'The good doctor', according to George D. LeMaitre, a Fellow of the American College of Surgeons,

> is much more than a well-trained technician or a scientist with a head full of facts. The practice of medicine remains, even in this scientific age, more art than science, more humanism than technology. Indeed there is much to suggest that science and technology have somehow perverted the art of medicine and dehumanized the physician. The decision to apply or misapply that technology is often a judgment of the heart rather than the head. Caring and curing cannot be separated. If you are looking for good scientific physicians, they are all around you. . . . But if you are looking for a good physician, one you can trust with your life and well being, start by looking for a human being who cares about you. (LeMaitre)

CHAPTER 6
The bodymind: mental influences

> The greatest discovery of my generation
> is that human beings may alter their lives
> by altering their attitude of mind.
>
> WILLIAM JAMES
> 1842–1910

One of the most serious deficits in second line medical practice, arising as it does out of the doctrine of specific etiology, is the failure to integrate into treatment a biological approach with a psychological one. George Engel, formerly Chairman of the Department of Psychiatry at the University of Rochester School of Medicine, has been perhaps the pre-eminent advocate of instituting a 'biopsychosocial' model into the practice of medicine. In a 1977 *Science* article, Engel proposed that,

> to provide a basis for understanding the determinants of disease and arriving at rational treatments and patterns of health care, a medical model must also take into account the patient, the social context in which he lives, and the complementary system devised by society to deal with the disruptive effects of illness, that is, the physician's role and the health care system (Engel, 1977).

Engel's proposal has not fallen upon deaf ears. Indeed, since the publication of his original article, Engel and others have expanded upon the importance of transforming the predominant medical model into one which straddles biological and psychological approaches (Engel, 1980; Swisher; Weiss). Despite a growing interest in the concept, however, the biopsychosocial model – just as the more controversial concept of holistic health – is unlikely to make a major impact upon medical practice in the immediate future. The institutions which have developed in the past century are so strongly predicated upon specific etiology doctrine (which Engel refers to as the 'biomedical model') that significant changes are a long way off.

Third Line Medicine, by contrast, has no need to struggle with the albatross of specific etiology doctrine; third line physicians already adhere to the ecologic, systems-oriented model which Engel has proposed. Their utilization of such a model, in fact, helps to explain why they may be capable of aiding patients who fail to benefit from first and second line interventions.

Previously, we have examined the origins of the current tension between ecologic models, such as Engel's, and the predominant 'biomedical' model, and we have explored the deleterious effects of rigid adherence to specific etiology doctrine within the modern practice of medicine. We shall now review the scientific evidence for eliminating the mind-body split which has plagued western medicine for many centuries. We will, at the same time, explore some of the integrative clinical techniques which are often utilized by third line physicians. These techniques are neither purely 'mental' nor 'physical', but are mental or physical approaches to what can best be called the 'bodymind'.

In this chapter, we shall examine the literature which supports the contention that *psychosocial* factors must be addressed in evaluating and treating illness; in the next chapter, we shall turn about to examine the literature which supports *physical* approaches to the treatment of illness. Both literatures are suggesting that figuratively splitting mind from body in dealing with a human being, instead of enabling health professionals to treat patients better, blinds these professionals from dealing with issues which have powerful effects upon the course of the illness. Together they form a powerful argument for fostering the growth and development of Third Line Medicine – at least until the entire institution of medical practice can be drastically overhauled to reflect the ecologic model.

One concept which has been particularly heuristic is that of psychosocial stress, defined by Z. J. Lipowski, Professor of Psychiatry at Dartmouth Medical School, as 'external and internal stimuli that are perceived by and are meaningful to the person, activate the emotions, and elicit physiologial changes that threaten health and survival.' (Lipowski) According to the experts, stress-related diseases are epidemic. Arnold Kadish, formerly Senior Research Associate at Caltech, for example, estimates that 80 per cent of the people who walk into doctors' offices are there because of stress-related diseases (Fryer); others estimate that between 75 and 90 per cent of illnesses are stress related (Brown). The only categories of illness not thought to be related to stress are those due to infection, injury, abnormal tissue activity or congenital birth defects.

Animal studies have provided much of the evidence of the link between stress and disease. In one study, for example, two monkeys were exposed for nine months to daily patterns of recorded noises comparable to those experienced by workers in the construction industry. The monkeys' hearing was not affected – but their blood pressure rose 27 per cent and stayed elevated for four months (Peterson).

Other animal studies have demonstrated that environmental stress is followed by an increase in tumor growth rates (La Barba). In one experiment, 92 per cent of mice placed under chronic stress developed mammary tumors, while 7 per cent of mice in a protected environment developed them (Riley).

Social isolation resulting in loneliness has been found to be one of the stress-producing factors which can lead to serious illness and even death. We know from animal studies that social contact even has a demonstrable effect on brain size. Young rats deprived of social contacts can lose up to 10 per cent of their brain size while, if old rats are put into a cage with young rats, the old rats' brains grow (Voss).

The *American Journal of Epidemiology* has published the results of a nine year Yale study which examined the relationship between social contact and health for a group of almost 5,000 men and women. The authors, Berkman and Syme, examined four different sources of social relationships: marriage, contacts with close friends and relatives, church or temple membership, and informal and formal associations with various clubs and organizations. They found that, 'in each instance', people with social ties and relationships had lower mortality rates than people without such ties. Each of the four sources was found to predict mortality independently of the other three; the more intimate ties of marriage and contact with friends and relatives were stronger predictors than were ties of church and group membership (Berkan and Syme).

The authors found that the men who were most isolated from others had a mortality rate 2.3 times greater than men with the most social connections; for women, the figure was 2.8 times higher. The more isolated people were, the more likely they were to die of heart disease, circulatory diseases, cancer, digestive and respiratory disturbances and even accidents (ibid.).

Other studies have found that a closely related factor, the loss of a spouse, has profound implications for health. The death rate for widows and widowers, for example, is ten times higher in the first year of bereavement than it is for others of comparable age. Similarly, in the year following divorce, the ex-spouses have twelve times the incidence of disease that married persons have (Knowles).

Conversely, a fascinating animal study has suggested that pleasant social interaction may offer protection from diet-induced arteriosclerosis (hardening of the arteries). Rabbits on a 2 per cent cholesterol diet were individually petted, held, talked to and played with on a regular basis while a control group on the same diet received the usual laboratory animal care. At the end of the experiment, the experimental group showed more than a 60 per cent reduction in aortic fat deposits compared to the control group (Nerem *et al.*).

Thomas H. Holmes and Richard H. Rahe of the Washington University School of Medicine in Seattle have constructed a Social Readjustment Rating Scale which has enabled researchers to undertake a more systematic approach to the investigation of the relationship between life stresses and various illnesses. The scale consists of forty-three items indicative of either the individual's lifestyle or of occurrences involving the individual. Each event has been assigned a relative value based on the degree to which it related to a significant change in the individual's ongoing life pattern (Holmes and Rahe, 1967).

Holmes and Rahe have administered the scale to over 5,000 subjects. Their findings: people who experienced significant elevations of life change units developed a variety of disorders in the succeeding year. These disorders included cancer, heart disease, multiple sclerosis, tuberculosis, skin disease and problem pregnancies as well as mental disorders and even injuries due to accidents. The severity of the disorder was correlated with the total score on the scale, especially in relation to chronic, stress-related illnesses. 37 per cent of those who scored from 150 to 200 in a twelve month period developed a serious ailment during that year. Those with scores of 200 to 300 had a better than even chance of becoming ill, while 80 per cent of those with scores of over 300 became ill (Holmes and Masuda).

The results of these studies suggest that the occurrence of psychologically stressful events bear a significant relationship to the subsequent manifestation of disease. As impressive as they are, they probably underestimate the extent of the relationship, since they fail to consider the established fact that individuals experience widely different amounts of stress from identical life events. We can expect, therefore, that individuals who, for constitutional or psychological reasons, are particularly prone to stress reactions will have an even greater likelihood of subsequent illness after exposure to stressors than that suggested by the data.

Evidence that the mental health of individuals, like the amount of psychological stress they are subjected to, is related to their subsequent physical health comes from an ongoing study at Harvard. The subjects are 204 men who have been followed since they were Harvard sophomores between 1942 and 1944. Of the men rated as having had the worst mental health between the ages of twenty-one and forty-six, 38 per cent had died or had become chronically ill by the age of fifty-three. By way of contrast, of the men rated as having had the best mental health during the same ages, only 3 per cent had died or had become chronically ill by the age of fifty-three. This link between previous mental health and subsequent physical health remained true regardless of the presence of other factors known to influence susceptibility to physical illness; namely, alcohol and tobacco use, weight, and the lifespan of the subjects' ancestors (Vaillant).

Samuel Silverman, a member of the clinical faculty at Harvard and a training analyst at the Boston Psychoanalytic

Institute, believes that he has isolated the specific individual characteristics which predict the imminent development of a physical illness through his study of data gathered during psychoanalysis. These include:

1 exposure to psychologic stress
2 a history of physical dysfunction as part of the general style of adaptation to psychologic stress
3 inadequate awareness and expression of relevant emotions
4 a persistent increase in awareness of physical sensations and perceptions
5 a morbid preoccupation with specific disturbances in close family friends.

Silverman believes that some of these characteristics provide clues, not only to the impending development of serious diseases, but also to the site or type of disease which is developing. He does not claim that these characteristics bear a causal relationship with the physical illness which later surfaces; rather he believes that they are very early signals of physical dysfunction (Silverman).

In September of 1974, Silverman was interviewed by *Time* magazine concerning his views on the effect of the Watergate scandal on President Nixon. He noted that 'Richard Nixon's target areas are the legs (phlebitis in 1964 and 1974, two knee injuries in 1960 and a foot injury in 1952) and the respiratory system (pneumonia in 1917 and 1973), with the ominous possibility that these two areas could be connected by a fatal blood clot traveling from leg to lung.' A further indication that the lungs could be involved was, according to Silverman, the death of Nixon's brother from pulmonary tuberculosis.

Only days after the interview, Richard Nixon was stricken with the blood clot in his lungs which Silverman had forecast, even though the chances against phlebitis leading to pulmonary embolism are five to one. Such fascinating predictions do not prove Silverman's hypothesis, but they do suggest that the link between the mind and body may be even more intimate than many have imagined. In another interview, Silverman has declared that 'I and others like me think that every illness, from the common cold to cancer, has a psychologic component – not an etiology but a component – for which we should be on the lookout.' (Leff)

Many other investigators have sought to identify the relationship between specific psychologic factors and specific diseases. While some of the proposed theories, such as Franz Alexander's specificity theory, have been largely discredited, others have been repeatedly confirmed. An example is the work of cardiologists Meyer Friedman and Ray Rosenman who noticed that patients developing coronary heart disease had certain personality features in common. Their investigations established that their observations were correct. They found that the coronary prone individual was likely to have a 'Type A' personality, the most relevant feature of which was a sense of incessant, unrelenting time pressure combined with 'the chronic struggle to grasp vaguely defined elements from the environment in the shortest period of time.' (Friedman and Rosenman)

Theories relating cancer to the mind go all the way back to Galen (200 AD) who stated that melancholic women developed breast cancer more often than did sanguine women. It may turn out that Galen was right. In a recent literature survey, Claus Bahne Bahnson, Professor of Psychiatry at Jefferson Medical College, concluded that,

> although there can be little doubt that a subtle relationship exists between loss and depression and the clinical onset or exacerbation of cancer, the question still remains whether some persons are more vulnerable than others because of their idiosyncratic way of responding to, or coping with, depression. (Bahnson)

Martin Seligman has suggested that depression can be studied in animals by employing a behavioral model. When an animal is subjected to repeated stressors from which it cannot escape, Seligman has shown that it eventually gives up trying to do so – and won't even attempt to escape once escape becomes possible. He calls this maladaptive behavior 'learned helplessness' and suggests it is the equivalent to what we experience as depression (Seligman).

With this model in mind, a recent study in *Science* seems to confirm the relationship between depression, i.e. 'learned helplessness', and cancer. Mice in whom tumor cells had been transplanted were subjected to electric shocks. Those who were unable to escape from the shock exhibited an earlier tumor appearance, larger tumor size and a decreased survival time (Sklar).

Not only have studies demonstrated a relationship between psychosocial factors and physical illness, but an increasing number of experiments have demonstrated biological mechanisms by which the mind may *provoke* bodily changes which, in turn, will cause the development of disease or even death. For example, death from heart attacks is usually attributed to reduction in the supply of oxygen to the heart (cardiac ischemia) due to atherosclerosis of the coronary arteries. This results in ventricular fibrillation (irregular and ineffectual contractions of the heart muscle) which is the direct cause of death. This simplistic explanation, which is characteristic of explanations based on specific etiology doctrine, fails to account for the fact that many victims of coronary atherosclerosis never develop ventricular fibrillation, or the fact that 15 per cent of those who die from fibrillation do not have coronary atherosclerosis (Skinner).

Walter B. Cannon, the famous Harvard physiologist, provided an explanation for these discrepancies back in 1931 by postulating the existence of a cerebral defense mechanism which, in emergency situations, took over from the lower brain stem centers which normally control the internal organs. Subsequent research has confirmed Cannon's hypothesis and located the cerebral defense mechanism in the frontal cortex. Animal studies have suggested that activating this area of the brain can lead to death from ventricular fibrillation even when the blood supply to the heart is sufficient. Conversely, these studies suggest that reduction of the blood supply to the heart will only produce fibrillation if the animal is stressed (ibid.).

It appears, therefore, that ischemia of the cardiac muscle predisposes an individual to death from ventricular fibrillation, but does not precipitate the event. Fibrillation occurs when the predisposed individual becomes emotionally stressed, and thus causes the cerebral defense mechanism to activate the neural pathways which initiate it.

Evidence has also been accumulating that psychosocial stress can provoke the brain to take measures which lessen the body's immune defenses. The implications of this line of research are staggering, since our protection from a broad range of diseases, from the common cold to cancer, is dependent upon the competence of the immune system. Immunosuppression has been found to occur, for example, in people grieving over the loss of their spouses (Bartrop *et al.*). One study performed at New York's Mount Sinai Hospital School of Medicine reported on men whose wives had just died of breast cancer. As early as two weeks after their wives' demise, the men showed a striking drop in the white cell response to stimulants of the immune system (*Medical World News* 21 July 1980). Such findings may explain the vastly increased death rate among widows and widowers alluded to earlier. Even the development of arteriosclerosis may be facilitated by means of stress-induced immunosuppression. In a study of laboratory rats published in *Science*, Rutgers researchers reported that the stress of multiple pregnancies was associated with the development of a type of immunological alteration conducive to arteriosclerosis. They suggested that 'this model of arteriosclerosis might be included in the same category of disorders as some autoimmune or viral conditions that manifest immune complex deposition in tissues as well as significant immune suppression.' (Lattime and Strausser)

Animal studies are also starting to reveal the biological mechanisms by which stress may lead to immunosuppression and thence to the development of diseases normally avoided by the healthy organism. Researchers at Johns Hopkins subjected a group of laboratory mice to loud noises for several days and then compared the state of their immune systems with those of mice that were not subjected to the noise. Their conclusion, reported in *Science*, was that immunosuppression due to stress is mediated through the action of cortisone, a steroid released from the adrenal gland, upon lymphocytes (cells which are key elements in immune responses) (Monjan and Collector). Vernon Riley has reached the same conclusion as a result of his own experiments which demonstrated that high levels of corticosteroids diminish immune functions which are restored when corticosteroid antagonists are injected (Riley).

Another mechanism by which the brain may influence the development of illness is by means of its manner of interpreting sensory stimuli. Researchers have found that the brain has a 'sensoristat' which tends habitually to augment sensory stimuli in some people – who are called 'augmentors' – and reduce them in others – who are called 'reducers'. Since augmentors have a different experience when exposed to the same stressors as reducers, they differ from reducers in their tendencies towards illness. Alcoholics, for example, are usually augmentors; alcohol tends to lessen their tendency to augment and thus may attract them for this reason. Augmentors are also more affected than reducers by painful stimuli, while reducers are less able to cope with situations which provide little sensory stimulation (Petrie, Buchsbaum).

A similar mechanism may alter our perception of specific stimuli on the basis of our emotional reaction to them. Stimuli which are aversive to the individual (annoying, fearsome, painful, etc.) tend to attract attention. The more attention they are given, the more intense the stimuli will appear to become. An example is the sound of a leaking faucet which, for our discussion, will represent an aversive stimulus. If you are in a room with a leaking faucet, but attending to something else, chances are that you would be unaware of the sound of the drip. If, however, you are starting to fall asleep in the same room, the sound of the drip will probably become apparent. The more you listen to it, and the more it bothers you, the louder it will seem.

Hypochondria refers to irrational fears of physical disease which can cause people to preoccupy themselves with worrisome bodily sensations. This process may reach the point where their fear incapacitates them. Cultural factors also influence the way we perceive and react to sensory stimuli. Researchers have found, for example, that different ethnic groups react differently to an electric shock (Sternbach and Tursky).

The emotions bridge mind and body. Their expression is both direct (as changes in the functional state of the body) and indirect (as expressed through language). In situations in which the indirect expression of emotions is reduced, their direct expression appears to be enhanced. The result is an increased tendency to develop pathologic physiochemical changes.

'Masked' emotions refer to emotions which are not acknowledged through language although there is both psychological and physiological evidence for their existence. The best studied of these has been masked depression which has been found to occur as often as does overt depression (Kielholz, Lesse). Masked anxiety is undoubtedly as common as masked depression, although it has received much less attention.

In 1967, Peter Sifneos coined the term 'alexithymia' to describe what is now considered to be a behavioral syndrome evidenced by many patients who are afflicted with psychosomatic illness (Sifneos). Alexithymics are unable to describe their feelings, even though they may be able to label them. They are also unable to relate feelings to their physiological expressions in their bodies and to distinguish between different feelings (Nemiah).

Much of our understanding of the relationship between the operations of the brain and illness continues to rest upon psychodynamic concepts which postulate that individuals may sometimes become ill in order to fulfill an emotional need. In other words, in certain instances people are less distressed when ill than when they are well. They may yearn to be taken care of and yet believe that, unless they are too ill to function, they must devote themselves to taking care of others' needs. The illness, then, both removes them from loathsome activities in a facesaving way and provides them with gratifications ranging from attention to financial rewards.

The anatomic source of the relationship between reason and emotion on one hand, and bodily changes on the other, can be traced to an area deep within the brain called the hypothalamus. It is a tiny region, located just above the pituitary gland, which consists of a number of cellular masses called the hypothalamic nuclei. It is closely connected with the cerebral cortex above it which not only performs the ultimate analysis of sensory data but also initiates motor impulses which, in turn, initiate, reinforce or inhibit the entire spectrum of muscular and glandular activity.

The hypothalamus is no less intimately connected with the deeper brain regions associated with emotions and the degree of activation of the bodily functions controlled by neurologic pathways. Finally, it is the supreme commander of the pituitary gland which resides beneath it. The pituitary, for its part, is the master gland for the regulation of glandular functions which are not controlled by neuronal pathways, with responsibilities over the adrenals, the thyroid, pancreas, and gonads. It also exercises direct control over water balance, blood pressure, body temperature, wakefulness and emotional behavior.

The key role of the hypothalamus in determining immunocompetence has been elucidated in an elegant series of studies from eastern Europe. A specific lesion produced in the hypothalamus was found to suppress the immune response to foreign proteins. On the other hand, electrical stimulation of the same site caused an immune response which was earlier, greater in magnitude and longer lasting than usual (Korneva).

It is thus incontrovertible that reason and emotion both influence and are influenced by complex regulatory mechanisms involving an enormous number of somatic activities. Since the brain has such powerful effects upon the functions of the rest of the body, we might expect that inadequate and maladaptive brain response to physical, chemical and psychic stressors could encourage and even initiate changes in the physiologic and biochemical activities of the organism, and that these changes could lead to the development of a wide variety of illnesses.

THE MIND AS A HEALING FORCE

If the brain can have a deleterious influence upon health, might it not be harnessed so as to expedite the process of healing? Neurochemists are making remarkable advances in influencing brain processes by changing the effective levels of neurotransmitters and other natural chemicals for which the brain has been found to have receptor sites. The implications of these advances for the treatment of major depressions, psychoses and certain neurologic syndromes have been widely recognized; however, their implications for the treatment of illnesses which are not considered to be primarily psychiatric or neurologic have been neglected. Similarly, endocrinologists are developing improved methods of affecting hypothalamic and pituitary functioning – but only applying them to the treatment of illnesses which can be attributed to gross abnormalities in the function of these structures.

With medical practice continuing to be dominated by specific etiologists, the possibility of utilizing the *normal* brain to influence the course of illnesses to which specific etiologies have been ascribed has been largely ignored. Psychiatry, of all the medical specialties, has come closest to examining this possibility, since the process of psychotherapy, although primarily applied to people identified as having a 'mental illness', seeks to combat illness by changing destructive mental processes and behaviors through the use of psychological interventions.

What is it about psychotherapy which provokes restorative processes? While psychiatry has been beset by numerous, and often contradictory, theoretical models, there have been no convincing demonstrations that any form of psychotherapy is superior to the others (Bergin and Lambert). On the other hand, a number of studies investigating the outcome of psychotherapy have shown that the manner in which psychiatrists relate to their patients, rather than the theory and techniques to which they subscribe, is the relevant variable in determining therapeutic effectiveness.

Charles Truax and Robert Carkhuff, for example, were able to demonstrate that psychotherapists who displayed three specific positive qualities in relating to their patients achieved better therapeutic results than those who did not. They characterized these qualities as genuineness or authenticity, empathic understanding and non-possessive warmth. Guided by their research results, they developed a training program which focused on the therapists' behavior towards their patients. With less than a hundred hours of training, these new therapists were able to achieve a level of effectiveness commensurate with that of experienced psychotherapists (Truax and Carkhuff). In a similar vein, Hans Strupp and Suzanne Hadley compared a group of highly experienced psychotherapists with a group of college professors chosen for their ability to form understanding relationships. Patients treated by the professors showed, on average, as much improvement as patients treated by the professional therapists (Strupp and Hadley).

Jerome Frank, Professor of Psychiatry Emeritus at Johns Hopkins, suggests that any positive psychotherapeutic influence contains the following features:

1 an intense, emotionally charged, confiding relationship with a helping person

2 a rationale, or myth, that includes an explanation of the cause of the patient's distress and that indirectly strengthens the patient's confidence in the therapist
3 provision of new information concerning the nature and sources of the patient's problems and possible alternative ways of dealing with them
4 strengthening the patient's expectations of help through the personal qualities of the therapist, i.e. the arousal of hope
5 provision of success experience that further heightens the patient's hope and enhances his sense of mastery and interpersonal competence
6 facilitation of emotional arousal. (Frank)

If psychosocial factors are relevant to the clinical course of all illnesses, not merely 'mental illnesses', might Hippocrates be correct in asserting that the relationship which patients have with their physicians can affect their clinical course? In that case, the features which Frank alludes to are as basic to the practice of medicine as are the contents of the physician's black bag.

Patients suffer *illnesses* (experiences of disvalued changes in states of being and social functioning) while specific etiologists diagnose and treat *diseases* (disturbances of the organs or body fluids characterized by structural alterations or chemical changes) (Kleinman *et al.*, Cassell). Illness is not necessarily associated with disease. Even when it is, similar degrees of structural pathology may generate widely different reports of pain and distress (Zola, Beecher). Also, the clinical course of an illness often differs from the course of the disease (Stoeckle *et al.*).

Patients seek treatment because they wish to be healed of their illnesses, not merely to be cured of their diseases. Thus, when physicians are disease-oriented specific etiologists, there is a fundamental difference between the goals of patients and the goals of their doctors. This difference helps to explain why an estimated 70 to 90 per cent of all episodes of illness are managed exclusively outside the formal health care system (Zola) as well as the shocking fact that patients report far greater improvement after treatment by folk healers than after treatment by modern physicians (Kleinman). It also helps to explain why patients often fail to comply with their doctors' orders (Stimson).

If, on the other hand, physicians join with their patients in a therapeutic alliance directed at the treatment of the *illness*, their effectiveness is vastly enhanced. Their responsibilities are considerably greater, since they can no longer content themselves with dealing with a dehumanized disease. Instead, they must also attempt to modify the psychosocial factors which contribute to the illness by stimulating their patients to examine their psychological position and to correct destructive tendencies.

Not only do third line physicians teach their patients how to make beneficial lifestyle changes, but they also train them in skills which augment their own abilities to modify their illnesses in the direction of healing. One of these skills is the ability to place the body in a state of relaxation.

It has long been common knowledge that relaxation has beneficial effects upon health. Over the centuries, a number of techniques emerged which promoted the attainment of a relaxed state of being. The eastern religions gave us Yoga and Zen meditation while the west developed hypnosis in the nineteenth century as well as progressive muscular relaxation and autogenic training in the twentieth. With the dawn of the modern scientific era, investigators began to document the actual changes in the functional state of the body which occurred during the performance of these techniques. While a large literature developed, each technique was studied alone, as if its effects were unique.

The fact that a variety of techniques could produce the same results was finally pointed out in a paper published in 1974 by Herbert Benson, Associate Professor of Medicine at Harvard Medical School, and two of his students (Benson). The authors reviewed the existing data on these techniques and showed that each could produce identical physiological changes. These changes they labeled 'the relaxation response'. The relaxation response, they stated, was controlled by the hypothalamus and was associated with decreased activity in the sympathetic nervous system, and possibly with increased activity in the parasympathetic nervous system (Benson *et al.*).

Benson's contribution was to give us a more scientific way of looking at activation of the autonomic nervous system and the procedures designed to affect it. Our nervous system is provided with two systems of controls over body movements. One system, which carries out our direct commands, is called the voluntary nervous system. The other system, in order to contrast it to the voluntary nervous system, is called the autonomic nervous system. 'Autonomic' means acting independently of volition. Until the late 1960s, the term seemed appropriate. Then our understanding of the way the autonomic nervous system operates radically changed.

This change was largely due to the work of Rockefeller Foundation scientist Neal Miller. Miller demonstrated that animals who were drugged so as to be unable to use the voluntary nervous system were still capable of being trained to make voluntary changes in the regulation of activities controlled by the autonomic nervous system. He produced these changes by rewarding the animals for making changes in a specific activity (such as heart rate) in the desired direction (Miller). His demonstration that the autonomic nervous system could be willfully controlled by providing biological feedback sent shock waves throughout the scientific community and spurred numerous studies on human subjects to see how well they could be trained to regulate functions normally controlled outside of their awareness or volition. The success of these studies changed our concepts of human capabilities and encouraged the development of clinical applications of biofeedback.

Like Miller's animal studies, clinical biofeedback procedures have focused on the provision of biological feedback as the device by which autonomic learning can be achieved. In these procedures, physiologic variables are utilized to provide people with information about the current functional state of their bodies. Feeling your pulse or observing your breathing pattern is thus a simple form of biofeedback. Many body functions are more difficult to observe, at least partly because we have never been taught how to become aware of them. For these functions, electronic equipment has been developed to change these subtle body signals in ways which help us to begin to appreciate them. Compact in size, but sophisticated in design, these instruments constantly monitor and amplify the desired physiologic signal much like the electrocardiograph (EKG) monitors the electrical signals being emitted by the heart.

Since physiologic signals often change so rapidly that they appear meaningless if we observe them just the way they occur, biofeedback instruments remove the confusing aspects of the signal and convey back to us just the amount of information which we can follow comfortably. Sometimes they convey the information by movements of a meter or on a strip chart just like other electronic medical instruments. Often they make changes in the physiologic activity still more observable and meaningful by converting the signal into flashing lights or sounds which change in pitch according to the strength of the signal.

In the past decade, numerous scientific studies have proven the effectiveness of biofeedback training of a single physiologic modality for a number of clinical applications (Gatchel and Price). Studies investigating applications of relaxation response training without the use of biofeedback have demonstrated that it is also an effective means of treatment (Benson). When one procedure is compared to the other, neither has been proven to be more effective (Silver and Blanchard). Combining the two procedures into biofeedback-assisted relaxation response training would appear to be the most potent manner of utilizing these treatments in a clinical setting – since biofeedback appears to expedite the learning of the relaxation response – although this hypothesis is still largely unproven (ibid.).

When the autonomic nervous system becomes overly activated, a number of common symptoms may be produced, including:

anxiety syndromes
cardiac arrhythmias
chronic pain syndromes
hypertension
insomnia
migraine headaches
muscle spasms
Raynaud's syndrome
spastic colitis
tension headaches
tinnitus

Relaxation response training, especially when assisted by the provision of biofeedback, provides people with a method of reducing these symptoms and healing themselves by learning to regulate their own bodies more effectively. Self-healing is far more preferable to drugs and surgery, since it utilizes the body's own regulatory mechanisms to initiate beneficial changes rather than forcing the body to accept such changes. In the latter case, these changes often stimulate the body's attempts to reject them, causing the development of adverse effects from the treatment. Other adverse effects are due to our inability to mimic natural processes with adequate precision.

In addition, since relaxation response training is a training program affecting the entire person, not merely the symptom, its benefits extend beyond symptom reduction. People going through the training and succeeding in improving their skills become more relaxed people. They are less irritable, less tense and anxious, and more able to cope with stressful situations. Just as their initial symptoms may be either psychologic (such as anxiety) or physical (such as irregular heart rhythm), the benefits of training encompass both aspects of their being. Moreover, the achievement of improvement by self-regulation generates a sense of self-satisfaction and pride, something which no medication or surgical procedure can ever provide.

Relaxation training provides yet another important benefit. We live in an achievement oriented culture which tends to view the body merely as a vehicle to be employed in order to attain goals. Third line patients, like many other people, thus fail to perceive the messages which their bodies send to indicate the corporal aspects of their feelings. The fact that the body is not an appendage to the mind but an integral part of the self is not often appreciated, nor is the fact that we can obtain as much information about the way we feel from our physical state as we can from our mental state.

Relaxation training first teaches people to become aware of body signals which indicate hyperactivation. In a sophisticated setting, the professional working with the patient then assists the patient in relating those signals to internal mental activity. In this manner, people can gradually learn to use changes in the functional state of their bodies as sources of information on their personal feelings and reactions. A result of such training is a substantial increase in self-awareness which assists people in making better decisions for themselves.

It is now generally accepted that, by means of procedures such as relaxation response training, people can learn to make beneficial physiologic changes – although the effect of these changes upon the eventual course of the illness is still debated. More controversial is the application of psychological procedures to the treatment of diseases marked by actual destruction of the body's tissues. So far, interest in this area has focused upon altering the course of cancer.

Spontaneous regression of cancerous tumors has been well documented (*Medical World News* 7 June 1974) but the reasons for such regressions have not been understood. For centuries there have been anecdotal reports of cancer regression through faith healing, but it has not been possible to ascertain whether the regression was, in fact, due to another coincident factor.

Carl Simonton, a radiologist, and his wife Stephanie, attempted to devise a program which would teach cancer patients to affect the course of their malignancies by utilizing their minds. Patients entered the program with the information that they would explore emotional factors as related to their health with the possibility of altering their clinical course. In addition to continuing their traditional medical treatments, they participated in a program of psychotherapy which included the use of guided imagery techniques as the central psychological exercise. Patients employed muscular relaxation and regular breathing while imagining specific scenes concerning such issues as their fears, childhood decisions and confronting the cancer in a symbolic fashion (Simonton *et al.*).

The Simontons found that the groups of patients so treated survived up to twice as long as would have been expected based on national averages for their respective cancers. They admit, however, that they remain uncertain at present as to the specific factors which account for the enhanced longevity of their patients (ibid.).

The direct effects of psychological factors upon illness have been characterized under the general term of 'placebo effects.' In contemporary western medicine, 'placebo' refers to a treatment which has no known effects of its own but still produces effects in the patient. The following definition, proposed by Cornell University Professor Arthur K. Shapiro, has become widely accepted:

> A placebo is any therapy, or component of therapy, that is deliberately or knowingly used for its nonspecific, psychologic, or psychophysiologic effect, or that is used unknowingly for its presumed or believed specific effect on a patient, symptom, or illness, but which, unknown to patient and therapist, is without specific activity for the condition being treated. (Shapiro)

Since the placebo effect is nonspecific and, moreover, cannot be described in physiologic or chemical language (Peek), specific etiologists have been biased against investigating it, and there has been little interest in developing methods of utilizing – and even enhancing – the effect for the benefit of patients. Indeed, research studies are routinely designed to evaluate if a specific treatment is more effective than the 'mere' placebo effect. Such studies disregard the fact that the benefits due to the effect are usually achieved with far less risk than the benefits of the specific treatment being studied.

Recent studies suggest that the placebo effect can indeed be explained, though in the language of psychology rather than in the language of physiology or chemistry. Richard Totman, for example, has proposed that the effect is due to cognitive dissonance (i.e. after people have made a decision, they will do things to justify it) (Totman). Ian Wickramasekera agrees that the effect can be explained in psychological terms, although he has proposed that it follows the model of Pavlovian conditioning (Wickramasekera).

Whatever its explanation, the placebo is the key to powerful internal forces. For example, Harvard anesthesiologist Henry K. Beecher reviewed fifteen studies of over a hundred patients and concluded that placebos reduce severe pain by 50 per cent in about one out of three patients (Beecher). A review of subsequent double-blind studies concluded that placebos are about half as powerful as whatever pain medication they are compared with, irrespective of how strong that medication is known to be in relieving pain (Evans).

Chronic pain is not the only medical condition which responds to placebos. Reports have been published in the medical literature claiming that placebos have successfully treated numerous ailments including:

- vascular disorders
  - ex. migraine headaches
    - strokes
    - hypertension
    - angina pectoris
    - intermittent claudication
- neurologic disorders
  - ex. Parkinsonism
    - multiple sclerosis
    - senile brain disease
- rheumatic disorders
  - ex. osteoarthritis
- allergies
  - ex. hay fever
    - asthma
- gastrointestinal disorders
  - ex. irritable bowel syndrome
- mental disorders
  - ex. neuroses
    - psychoses
- skin disorders
  - ex. warts
    - acne
- endocrine and metabolic disorders
  - ex. menopausal symptoms
    - diabetes mellitus
    - obesity
- sleep disorders
  - ex. insomnia (Totman)

Until fairly recently, the anti-placebo bias caused physicians to assume that placebos merely deluded patients with physical diseases into believing that they were better while the course of the disease remained unaltered. Now scientific investigations are discovering that placebos produce definite changes in biological processes. It appears, for example, that placebos relieve the experience of pain by stimulating the release of endorphins (endogenous morphine-like substances) in the brain. Morphine and other narcotics are now known to relieve pain by fooling endorphin receptors in the brain into responding to their presence as if they were true endorphins (Levine).

Due to the influence of specific etiologists, there is a recurring theme in the medical literature that, since placebos are nonspecific, people who respond to them are being deluded and therefore are more gullible and less mentally fit than those who do not. This is despite the fact that careful studies have failed to find any relationship between placebo responsiveness and gullibility or suggestibility (Evans). Other studies have established that intelligence is directly correlated to response to placebos (Gold). A Mayo Clinic study has found that the tendency to respond to placebos was correlated to years of education and job skills, and that placebo responders shared a way of life that demanded responsibility, self-sufficiency, and independent work; yet the authors still hypothesized that the placebo response may be a type of hypnosis resulting from 'exaggerated oral-dependency needs!' (Moertel)

A double-blind study published in the *Journal of Psychosomatic Research* has clarified some of the issues. People relatively free of emotional problems ('Normals') were compared to people who were physically tense and psychologically rigid ('Hypernormals') and emotionally troubled people ('Psychoneurotics'). When placebos were given in a neutral manner (as is usual in drug studies), Normals were most responsive to placebo effects (53 per cent), with Hypernormals in the middle (33 per cent) and Psychoneurotics the least responsive (14 per cent). When, however, placebos were given with strong positive assurances that they would be effective, Normals became less responsive, while both Hypernormals and Psychoneurotics became more responsive. The result was that Psychoneurotics were now the most responsive group (69 per cent), with Hypernormals in the middle (50 per cent) and Normals the least responsive (36 per cent) (Shipman *et al*).

The placebo effect, therefore, has at least two components. The first is suggestion. This component is communicated exclusively through the medium of language. The second component is a physical ritual performed by or upon the patient. In modern guise, the ritual is usually the swallowing of a pharmacologically inert capsule or the performance of surgery upon the patient.

The tremendous power of the physical ritual was demonstrated by a study reported in the *Archives of General Psychiatry*. Instead of the usual procedure of deluding patients into believing that placebos are powerful drugs, fifteen psychoneurotics agreed to try what they knew to be a dummy pill. After one week of such treatment, improvement was assessed by means of both a clinical examination and the patients' own ratings of their symptoms. Fourteen of the fifteen patients returned for reassessment, and *all* of them had improved (Park and Cori)! Without a control group, we cannot know how much better they did than patients who were just asked to return one week later without having had to perform any ritual; however, the universal improvement in the patients who returned certainly suggests that the ritual itself had a powerful effect.

The value of the placebo lies in its capacity to harness the enormous healing power of the mind. Ultimately, it provides us with a means of utilizing our own resources. *We* are the real power of the placebo; the placebo is merely a device which assists us in using our abilities to heal ourselves when we are unable to read the roadmap unassisted. In the words of Albert Schweitzer (as quoted by Norman Cousins): 'Each patient carries his own doctor inside him. We are at our best when we give the doctor who resides within each patient a chance to go to work.' (Cousins)

CHAPTER 7
The bodymind: physical influences

Disease is the retribution of outraged Nature.

HOSEA BALLOU
1771–1852

Just as the mind can be utilized to intervene in a manner which affects the course of illness in both its physical and psychological dimensions, a variety of physical interventions can influence the course of illness in both dimensions. The third line approach thus includes procedures designed to affect the illness by creating a salutary physical change in the body in as natural a manner as possible.

Many of these procedures involve educating patients as to the influence of their personal behaviors upon their health. Thomas McKeown, Professor of Social Medicine Emeritus at the University of Birmingham in England, asserts that, while nutrition, protection from hazards and population control have been, and will continue to be, major factors in determining health, personal behavior has now become a factor of greater importance (McKeown). This category includes such items as diet, exercise, and the use of drugs such as tobacco and alcohol.

For example, N.B. Belloc and Lester Breslow of UCLA studied the personal behaviors of 7,000 adults for five and a half years and found seven factors to be significantly related to life expectancy and health:

1 three regular meals daily with no snacking
2 daily breakfast
3 moderate exercise two or three times a week
4 seven to eight hours of sleep nightly
5 no smoking

6 moderate weight
7 no alcohol or alcohol only in moderation

Belloc and Breslow found that forty-five-year-old men who practiced at least six of these seven behaviors lived an average of eleven years longer than those who practiced three or less. This striking difference in life expectancy as related to personal habits contrasts with the fact that, between 1900 and 1966, only 2.7 years were added to the life expectancy of a person who had lived to age sixty-five (Belloc and Breslow).

Further evidence of the association between harmful personal habits and disease has come from a pair of Harvard investigators. They reviewed the records of over 2,000 people admitted to six hospitals and divided them into a high cost and a low cost group. The high cost group, while only 13 per cent of the patients, used as much of the hospital resources as the other 87 per cent. When they compared the two groups, they found that harmful lifestyles (particularly alcoholism, overeating and heavy smoking) were noted more often in the records of the high cost group. The high cost was largely due to the need for repeated hospitalizations which were not as common for those in the low cost group (Zook and Moore).

Given studies like these, experts are now estimating that as much as *80 per cent* of all deaths due to cardiovascular disease and cancer are 'premature;' that is, occur in relatively young individuals and are related to those individuals' bad habits (Knowles). Moreover, if health care services were more oriented towards prevention, research has shown that many of these premature deaths could be prevented. For example, on the basis of current data, it has been estimated that, if males between the ages of thirty-five and sixty-four participated in a program of risk factor intervention and lifestyle modification, 45 per cent of the present incidence of arteriosclerotic cardiovascular disease could be prevented (Marmot and Winkelstein).

Given the relatively nominal expense of providing such a program, the savings on the subsequent cost of medical services would be enormous. Unfortunately, first and second line physicians, guided by the doctrine of specific etiology, direct their energies primarily towards repairing the damage done by these destructive behaviors, while virtually neglecting the more important tasks of motivating patients to change destructive behaviors and teaching them how to do so.

This chapter will explore in detail some of these physical influences upon health, influences which third line physicians can harness to provoke healing processes by encouraging patients to expose themselves to them when they are healthy, and remove themselves from them when they are not.

NUTRITION AND HEALTH

> Let thy food be thy medicine
> and thy medicine be thy food.
>
> HIPPOCRATES (460–377 BC)

> No illness which can be treated by diet
> should be treated by any other means.
>
> MOSES MAIMONIDES (1135–1204 AD)

Few of the areas of medical research present such obstacles for the serious inquirer who wishes to gain a balanced perspective as does the area of clinical nutrition. At one end are the studies cited by the enthusiasts, usually in lay magazines, which suggest that many of the afflictions of the average 'well nourished' American can be prevented or cured by dietary manipulations. At the other end are the studies cited by the skeptics, usually in professional journals, which suggest that Americans are being seduced by the enthusiasts into food faddism which, at best, is a waste of money and, at worst, is downright dangerous. While the truth is doubtless somewhere in between, the skeptics commonly take the position that the claims of the enthusiasts are usually unsupported by scientific evidence. This is indeed the case; however, the results of recent studies have been lending increasing support to some of the enthusiasts' most cherished claims.

Any discussion of nutrition should start with an examination of the Recommended Dietary Allowances (RDAs) published by the Food and Nutrition Board of the National Academy of Sciences and available from the US Government Printing Office

(National Academy of Sciences). The RDAs are defined as:

> the levels of intake of essential nutrients considered, in the judgment of the Committee on Dietary Allowances of the Food and Nutrition Board on the basis of available scientific knowledge, to be adequate to meet the nutritional needs of practically all healthy persons.

These recommendations are of tremendous value to community planners as they provide a basis for designing dietary programs which meet minimal standards for the prevention of nutritional deficiency diseases.

Unfortunately professionals have been taught by the skeptics to treat the RDAs as dogma and to utilize them in situations in which they are not applicable. When the Food and Nutrition Board states that the RDAs meet the nutritional needs of 'practically all healthy persons', it is referring to its decision to set RDAs at a level which is adequate for approximately 97 per cent of the population and thus insufficient for the remaining 3 per cent. Since there are at least forty essential nutrients with a 3 per cent risk of deficiency for each, the risk that the RDA will be insufficient in one or more nutrients for a particular normal individual becomes substantial. In other words, if you ingest exactly the RDA of each nutrient, you are probably going to become deficient in at least one of them. As pointed out by the authoritative *Heinz Handbook of Nutrition*, 'the typical individual is more likely to be one who has average needs with respect to many essential nutrients, but who also exhibits some nutritional requirements for a few essential nutrients which are far from average.' (Burton)

Roger Williams has long argued that group norms conceal the biochemical individuality of each member of the group. Gio B. Gori, Deputy Director of the National Cancer Institute's Division of Cancer Cause and Prevention, agrees:

> The average American does not exist. We have a hypothetical average American, but the fact is that our country is made up of over 200 million individuals. Each one has his or her own specific requirements dependent on somatic characteristics, sex, age, amount of work and exercise, behavioral characteristics, type of personality,

> genetic characteristics, place of residence, etc. All these things impose variations on the daily nutrient requirements. One of the greatest challenges, in my opinion, in the next ten or twenty years is precisely this: to attempt to define the ranges of variability of personal intake of nutrients. . . . The plain and ugly truth is that we really do not know enough to establish individual, personal daily allowances because we have little grasp of the personal, individual variation in dietary requirements. (*Journal of the Nutritional Academy* October 1979.)

Not only may the typical individual be deficient in a few essential nutrients while ingesting the RDAs, but according to an article which appeared in *Nutrition Today*, 'there is some reason to believe that many people are falling significantly short of their RDA levels for vitamins and minerals.' (Scala) For example, in the Ten State Nutrition Survey conducted by the Department of Health, Education and Welfare of the United States Government (1968–70), which investigated the diets of adolescents and the elderly, approximately half the people surveyed were deficient in their intakes of calcium, iron, vitamin A, thiamin, riboflavin and vitamin C; in the Health and Nutrition Examination Survey (1971–4), also conducted by HEW, 93 per cent of the women surveyed who were between the ages of eleven and sixty were failing to ingest the RDA of iron.

Even if we assume that John Doe, by regularly ingesting 100 per cent of the RDAs of essential nutrients, will be able to avoid any signs or symptoms of the classical deficiency diseases, a considerable body of research data suggests that he will still be courting trouble. The Food and Nutrition Board states that:

> for certain nutrients the requirements may be assessed as the amount that will just prevent failure of a specific function or the development of specific deficiency signs – an amount that may differ greatly from that required to maintain maximum body stores.

A number of studies have shown that doses of nutrients far above the RDAs have additional effects beyond those examined by the Board. For example, Cheryl Nockels and her colleagues at Colorado State University fed one group of laboratory animals a diet which supplied the RDAs. A second group was given the identical diet except for additional vitamin E. In a series of experiments with a number of different animals, Nockels was repeatedly able to demonstrate that the group which received the additional vitamin E had superior resistance to infections (Nockels).

Man-Li Yew has reported on a similar experiment in which he found that the level of vitamin C required to optimize wound healing, promote the growth rate and reduce recovery time after anesthesia in guinea pigs was ten times higher than the amount required to prevent scurvy – the classical disease caused by vitamin C deficiency and prevented by ingesting the RDA of vitamin C. He concluded that:

> for young people the need is 20 times higher than the accepted Recommended Dietary Allowance. Individual needs vary over a wide range, and the implications of these findings may be much more widespread than just Vitamin C itself. (Yew)

Yet another deficit of using the RDAs or, for that matter, any arbitrary yardstick for determining nutritional status by measuring the level of ingested nutrients, is their failure to deal with the individual differences in tissue levels of nutrients when identical amounts are ingested. The assumption that such differences do not exist presupposes that individuals do not differ in the efficacy of the digestive processes which prepare the food for passage through the gut lining in the blood stream. It also presupposes that, once food is digested, all individuals are capable of comparable degrees of nutrient absorption. These are complex processes, and it is becoming increasingly doubtful that such facile assumptions can be made (Williams).

It should also be noted that of the fifty or so nutrients, only the minority have been assigned RDA levels. Research data on the others have so far been inadequate to establish RDAs; thus diets which are adequate in the known RDAs may still be deficient in a number of nutrients according to RDA criteria yet to be established.

Finally, the RDAs are only relevant to the nutritional requirements of healthy people. The Food and Nutrition Board notes that:

> special needs for nutrients arising for such problems as . . . inherited metabolic disorders, infections, chronic diseases and the use of medications require special dietary and therapeutic measures. These conditions are not covered by the RDA.

In other words, the RDA is meaningless as a measure of nutritional adequacy when applied to a population of medical patients, as these patients may well be suffering from nutritional deficits even though their diets meet the RDA for each essential nutrient.

To summarize, the Recommended Dietary Allowances provide valuable guidelines to assist investigators and planners in the field of public health. Their utility as a means of assessing nutritional adequacy for specific people, however, is quite limited. Evidence is accumulating that an individual's nutritional adequacy can be better assessed by using laboratory methods. The best of these, when available, are tests which, instead of comparing the individual to group norms, assess the functional adequacy of nutrients for the specific person being evaluated. For the clinician who recognizes that marginal nutritional deficiencies may provoke clinically significant signs and symptoms, the data provided by such studies are far more relevant to diagnosis and treatment than are the RDAs.

Another battleground between enthusiasts and skeptics has been the extent of the nutritional contribution to diseases other than the classical nutritional deficiency diseases. There is no question that, as the scientific literature in this area has grown, the skeptics have been rapidly losing ground to the enthusiasts. The evidence is now overwhelming, for example, that diet plays a major role in the development and progression of atherosclerotic cardiovascular disease, the single most common cause of death from disease in our society. Numerous studies have demonstrated that high levels of cholesterol, particularly low density lipoprotein cholesterol (LDL), are a major risk factor which occurs frequently in individuals with the disease, while high levels of triglycerides, low levels of high density lipoproteins (HDL) and obesity are secondary risk factors. Mary Winston, Chief of the American Heart Association's nutrition programs, notes that there is substantial evidence that all four of these risk factors can be modified by changes in dietary habits; plasma cholesterol, for example, appears to be largely determined by the intake of dietary cholesterol, saturated fat, polyunsaturated fat and calories (Winston).

Eating habits also appear to exert an influence on the development of cancer, the second most frequent cause of death. While current knowledge about the relationship between diet and heart disease is based on six decades of evidence, our knowledge about the relationship between diet and cancer is largely based on studies performed in the past decade. A recent governmental study states that diet may account for 35 per cent of all cancer mortality in the United states ('Avoidable risks'). Similarly, a National Research Council panel, after reviewing 10,000 reports in the literature, has concluded that the evidence is 'increasingly impressive that the cancers of most major common sites are influenced by dietary patterns.' (Horwitz)

One of the major dietary factors which correlates with the incidence of cancer is the level of dietary fat. Rates for bowel and breast cancer are much lower in Japan, where only 20 per cent of an average person's calories comes from fat – half the percentage of fat in the average American diet (*Medical World News* 17 October 1977). Unsaturated fats, which some experts have advocated because they appear to have a protective role in heart disease by lowering plasma cholesterol, are even worse than saturated fats in causing cancer in experimental animals (*Los Angeles Times* 26 November 1981); this may explain why very low levels of plasma cholesterol are correlated with an increased incidence of cancer (Cheraskin and Ringdorf).

Even more important than the percentage of dietary fat is a person's total calorie intake. 'By and large', states the National Cancer Institute's Gio B. Gori, 'animals that are fed a calorie-restricted diet develop fewer tumors and, on top of that, live much longer than animals that are fed with high-calorie daily intakes.'. (*Journal of the Nutritional Academy*) He suggests that, simply, on the basis of what we now know about the relationship between overeating and both heart disease and cancer,:

> it would seem prudent to reduce calories. In order to reduce calories, it would seem reasonable to suggest the

> reduction of those components of food that contribute the greatest amount of calories and the greatest amount of empty calories, those not contributing nutrients. These are fats, which are almost twice as calorific as the nearest thing, and sugar. We should increase roughage and fresh vegetables and fruit, which will not only increase the intake of fiber, but also the intake of minerals and vitamins and all the other micro-nutrients that seem to be so important (ibid.).

Scientific medicine is just beginning to appreciate the influence of nutrients upon the state of the mind. While medical students continue to be taught that nutritional deficiencies only exist in cases of severe malnutrition, investigators are finding such deficiencies to be surprisingly common among the mentally ill. For example, members of the Department of Psychiatry at McGill University divided forty-eight patients into three groups – depressed patients, psychiatrically ill but nondepressed patients, and medically ill patients. All were hospitalized for one week during which they received standard diets with no drugs or vitamins. At the end of this time, the depressed patients had significantly lower levels of serum folic acid than did the patients in the other two groups (Ghadirian *et al.*).

A deficiency of vitamin B 12 is also associated with mental symptoms. An editorial in *The Lancet* states that, in cases of B 12 deficiency, 'frank psychoses have been reported in between 4 per cent and 16 per cent of patients taking all forms from confusional states to affective conditions, although several workers note a tendency to paranoid symptoms' (*The Lancet* 25 September 1965). Vitamin B12 deficiency is commonly diagnosed on the basis of the development of pernicious anemia, a diagnosis which is readily apparent from routine blood studies. Most first and second line physicians, confident that such blood studies will provide the diagnosis, are unaware that the mental symptoms of the disease may precede any changes in the blood by several years (ibid.).

Another line of research exploring the relationship between nutrients and mental illness is investigating the effects of giving unnaturally high levels of particular nutrients to psychiatric patients who show none of the traditional clues to nutritional deficiencies. This approach has been called 'orthomolecular psychiatry' by two-line Nobel prize winner Linus Pauling. Though the effectiveness of orthomolecular approaches to schizophrenia has generated tremendous controversy (*Task Force Report* 7, Pauling), the possibility of utilizing unphysiologic doses of nutritional precursors of brain neurotransmitters has received early validation in a number of studies. For example, choline, the precursor of acetylcholine, may have beneficial effects in senile dementia (Boyd *et al.*). Tryptophan, precursor of serotonin, may have beneficial effects in insomnia (Hartman) and depression (Rao and Broadhurst), while tyrosine, precursor of norepinephrine, may be beneficial in depression (Gelenberg *et al.*). Research on the use of neurotransmitter precursors is preliminary, but their apparent safety argues for their use with selected patients.

Third line patients, with their typical histories of chronic illness, the use of multiple medications and lack of appetite, often suffer from the effects of nutritional inadequacies and imbalances. Even those with good diets may have nutritional deficits due to improper digestion, absorption or assimilation of nutrients, so a simple tally of what patients ingest will often give misleading data. For that reason, third line physicians seek to assess nutritional status by forms of testing which evaluate whether patients are receiving adequate nutrients for their individual needs. This is a far more important question than the one asked in first and second line medicine (that is, if any question concerning nutrition is even asked) which is whether they are ingesting the Recommended Dietary Allowances. Jonathan V. Wright, a nutritionally-oriented physician whose 'Prevention Clinics' appear regularly in *Prevention*, has summarized the conditions in which he believes nutritional therapy is likely to be beneficial:

> I've watched numerous circulatory problems improve, including return of ulcerated bluish-black feet and lower legs to normal color. Diabetes mellitus of varying severity can usually be improved, even 'cured,' as can high blood pressure. Complications of both illnesses can be prevented. The list of problems that can reasonably be expected to

improve with nutritional-biochemical therapy is long:
gallbladder disease
prostate problems
depression
eczema
bursitis
arthritis (many forms)
cystic mastitis
kidney stones
gout
anemia
colitis
premenstrual difficulties
toxemia of pregnancy
headache
infections
and more. That is only a small part of the list. . . . Nutritional-biochemical therapy may not always apply, or be best, but should always be considered before final decisions are made. (Wright)

RECREATIONAL DRUGS

Some of the most dreadful mischiefs
that afflict mankind proceed from wine;
it is the cause of disease, quarrels,
sedition, idleness, aversion to labour,
and every species of domestic disorder.

François de Salignac
de la Mothe Fenelon
1651–1715

The wretcheder one is,
the more one smokes;
and the more one smokes
the wretcheder one gets
– a vicious circle!

George Louis Palmella
Busson du Maurier
1834–96

Foods may at times have mind-altering effects, but recreational drugs are brought into the body specifically for the powerful effects they have upon a person's mental state. Society has had an ambivalent attitude towards these drugs, on the one hand condemning and sometimes outlawing them for their adverse effects, on the other hand supporting their use as an acceptable means of coping with burdensome stresses and distresses. Although the use of tobacco has been slowly declining, 32 per cent of adults continue to smoke (1982 Surgeon General's Report), and the average American smoker smokes 10.7 cigarettes a day (US Census Bureau). We now know that men who smoke are twice as likely as non-smokers to die of cancer, while women face a 30 per cent greater risk. In fact, 30 per cent of all deaths due to cancer can be attributed to cigarette smoking. Cancer, however, accounts for less than half of the deaths caused by smoking. The other deaths are due to heart disease, lung and respiratory diseases and other illnesses. In addition, smoking has been implicated in miscarriages, premature births and birth defects (op. cit.).

Perhaps even more destructive is alcoholism, since the behavioral effects of alcohol make inebriates dangerous, not only to themselves, but also to the rest of society. It has long been known that alcohol has an adverse effect on the heart muscle but, until recently, it was believed that this was due to the effect of liver disease which was caused by the alcohol. We now know that alcohol can weaken the heart muscle even if there is no liver disease and, in fact, alcoholic heart disease is a common abnormality (*Medical World News* 26 February 1971). In one study, a survey was made of the employees of a large industrial firm who were known or suspected problem drinkers. Compared to a group of non-alcoholic employees, they had a higher incidence of heart disease, hypertension, cirrhosis of the liver, stomach ulcer, duodenal ulcer, asthma, diabetes, gout, neuritis, and strokes (ibid.).

There is even some early evidence that the use of alcohol may double the risk of breast cancer, the most common form of cancer in women. According to one recent study, women who drank at least four days a week had 2 to 3½ times the risk of non-drinkers of getting breast cancer (Rosenberg *et al.*). While the possibility remains that this correlation was due to other factors, it suggests that we have yet to discover the full range of diseases promoted by alcohol ingestion.

Undoubtedly, there are a number of mechanisms by which alcohol usage promotes the development of illness. Alcohol is a high calorie food of negligible nutritional value which tends to replace the intake of quality foodstuffs. When it becomes the main source of calories, serious nutritional deficiencies may occur. Cirrhosis of the liver results from inadequate protein and lipotropics, brain damage and polyneuropathy from thiamine deficiency, and pellagra, a classical vitamin deficiency disease, from a deficiency of niacin. Alcohol also appears to have a direct effect on blood flow in small vessels, causing them to clog so that the flow of oxygen and nutrients to the cells is impeded (Moskow *et al.*).

Tobacco also promotes illness by a number of mechanisms. Respiratory diseases are encouraged by its destructive effect on the cilia (*The Health Consequences*). These are hairlike filaments which line the tubing of the lung and protect it from toxic substances. Tobacco smoke contains several chemicals which have carcinogenic activity. Since the gaseous phase of cigarette smoke contains about 4 per cent of carbon monoxide, the tissues of smokers are robbed of oxygen (ibid.). Nutritional mechanisms may also be involved. One study, for example, showed that smokers who take as much vitamin C as non-smokers have significantly lower serum levels of vitamin C (Pelletier).

Third line physicians often find that, not only do their patients frequently drink excessively or smoke, but that their first and second line physicians have neglected to educate them as to the relationship between their illnesses and their use of recreational drugs. For example, according to an article in *The New England Journal of Medicine*, 'the antismoking efforts of physicians . . . have been spotty and inconsistent.' (Brody) Small wonder that, even though physicians know enough to stop smoking themselves, the Federal Trade Commission has found that 25 per cent of heavy smokers don't even know that smoking is hazardous, 40 per cent don't know that it causes most lung cancer, and 60 per cent don't know that it causes most emphysema (Frederick).

Thus, in dealing with third line patients, third line physicians review their use of recreational drugs, educate them as to the relationship between drug use and their illnesses and suggest methods to them which may help them to modify their lifestyles so that they can cope with stresses without relying on such perilous substances.

EXERCISE AND HEALTH

Better to hunt in Fields, for Health unbought,
Than fee the Doctor for a nauseous Draught.
The wise, for Cure, on exercise depend;
God never made his Work, for Man to mend.

JOHN DRYDEN
1631–1700

The association between regular exercise and good health has long been a part of popular wisdom. Only recently, however, has medical science begun to confirm their relationship. The most sophisticated studies have concerned the relationship between aerobic conditioning and cardiovascular disease. In a recent editorial, *The New England Journal of Medicine* commented that 'it is no longer difficult to accept the fact that exercise has a direct and favorable association with processes important to cardiovascular health.' (Paffenbarger and Hyde) One of the mechanisms by which exercise exerts its effect is by influencing the metabolism of fats, since we now know that increased exercise leads to lower concentrations of triglycerides, very-low-density lipoprotein cholesterol (VLDL) and low-density lipoprotein cholesterol (LDL), while increasing concentrations of high-density lipoprotein cholesterol (HDL) (ibid.).

Another mechanism by which exercise may improve cardiovascular health is by enhancing fibrinolysis, the body's mechanism for dissolving dangerous blood clots. Researchers at Duke University exercised a group of healthy volunteers three times a week for ten weeks. The program consisted of ten minutes of stretching followed by thirty to forty-five minutes of walking or jogging. At the end of the program, most showed evidence of increased anticlotting ability, with those whose cholesterol levels were highest at the start of the experiment showing the greatest improvement (Williams *et al.*). These findings suggest that exercise protects, not merely against atherosclerotic heart disease, but also against all illnesses caused by blood clots – such as strokes, pulmonary emboli (blood clots from leg veins which travel to the lungs) and intermittent claudication (leg pains upon walking due to decreased arterial circulation).

Twenty years ago, few doctors recommended that diabetics risk the metabolic effects of regular exercise. We now know, however, that mild exercise lowers blood sugar and reduces the need for insulin. These effects appear to be due to an increase in insulin binding at the cellular level. It has been demonstrated that exercise increases the binding of insulin to red and white blood cells; increased binding in liver and muscle cells may also occur (Yates).

Aerobic exercise is the most beneficial. This is the form of exercise during which the oxygen demand of the muscles does not exceed the supply, as in constant but not overly strenuous activity. Anerobic exercise occurs when the oxygen demand exceeds the supply – as in brief periods of high exertion – and does not appear to be as effective (Auersbacher). Several months of regular practice is required to achieve major effects.

A frequent complaint of third line patients is chronic pain, and exercise is an important modality of treatment for many pain syndromes which is often neglected. Back pain is the single most common pain complaint. In one study, a combined medical group from New York and Columbia Universities evaluated 5,000 consecutive back pain patients and found that 81 per cent of them had pain due to muscular deficiency caused by inadequate physical activity (Friedmann).

The beneficial effects of exercise are not limited to its effects upon the body. Investigators have demonstrated that exercise can also benefit our emotional state. For example, Herbert deVries, Director of the Physiology of Exercise Laboratory at the University of Southern California, has found evidence that as little as twenty minutes of moderate exercise such as walking or cycling relieves tension and anxiety. In one study, the electrical activity of volunteers' muscles was tested for both immediate and chronic effects of exercise. Significant reductions in neuromuscular activity levels were found *(Clinical Psychiatry*

News January 1982).

Studies have also found that exercise has an anti-depressant effect. People who are essentially healthy but score in the depressed range on questionnaries note improved moods after exercise programs. In order to see if depressed psychiatric patients would also feel better after exercise, researchers at the University of Wisconsin studied a group of people who were diagnosed as depressed. Patients were randomly assigned either to a program of running or to one of two kinds of individual psychotherapy. At the end of ten weeks, six of the eight patients who ran had recovered from their depressions, a result comparable to the best outcomes obtained by psychotherapy for patients in their clinic (Griest *et al.*).

In Third Line Medicine, assessment includes evaluating the patient's state of physical fitness and the possible interaction between that state and the presenting illness. After educating the patient about the relationship between health and exercise, an exercise program is frequently recommended which, most importantly, is specifically tailored to both the patient's needs and level of motivation.

ACUPUNCTURE

> This is the way of acupuncture:
> if man's vitality and energy
> do not propel his own will
> his disease cannot be cured.
>
> THE YELLOW EMPEROR'S CLASSIC OF INTERNAL MEDICINE
> *c.* 300 BC

Since so much of the recent interest in acupuncture in the west has been focused on the treatment of pain, few people are aware that acupuncture is actually a complete system of medicine. In fact, it is the oldest surviving medical system in the world. Although its earliest origins are unknown, many of its concepts were systematized by 5,000 years ago. By the third century BC, the oldest known medical treatise, *The Yellow Emperor's Classic of Internal Medicine*, summarized the methods of acupuncture which had become standard practice.

There was little interest in acupuncture in the United States until 1971 when James Reston, a reporter for the *New York Times*, developed appendicitis while following President Nixon on his trip to China and was treated successfully with acupuncture for post-appendectomy pain. Physicians and journalists on the trip were also shown surgical operations using acupuncture for analgesia and returned with glowing accounts. Acupuncture rapidly became the newest medical fad, with numerous people suffering from all types of pain seeking out the treatment from anyone who would offer it.

The scientific community, meanwhile, while curious, was understandably skeptical. Early demonstrations of acupuncture analgesia for surgical procedures in this country confirmed its efficacy. The obvious question, however, was whether acupuncture was merely a form of hypnosis – since hypnosis had already been found to be effective in causing sufficient analgesia for a number of surgical procedures to be performed with comfort (Kroger). Besides, the explanation for the pain-relieving effect postulated the existence of a system of meridians through which 'energy' was said to flow. This system was unsubstantiated by modern anatomical knowledge and was totally foreign to the western system of medicine.

On the other hand, acupuncture was effective in relieving distress for two groups of subjects who were entirely unaware of why they were being stuck with the tiny needles – namely, animals and infants. If acupuncture was effective in naive subjects, there had to be something more to it than hypnosis. Thus, numerous research projects were undertaken in an effort to explain the effects of acupuncture in terms understandable to westerners.

One explanation has since been provided by Ronald Melzack of McGill University and his associates who noted that most acupuncture points (71 per cent) are identical to known trigger points (Melzack *et al.*). Trigger points are points of exquisite tenderness which may exist either within the painful area or distant from it. The degree of their tenderness bears a direct relationship to the degree of pain and their proper stimulation can lead to relief from pain due to muscular spasms (Travell and Rinzler).

Since trigger points had already been utilized in the treatment of pain syndromes for many years, their coincidence with acupuncture points provided an explanation for the effects of acupuncture which made the procedure more acceptable to western physicians. This was despite the fact that the nature of trigger points is not entirely understood.

It was a biochemical explanation for acupuncture's pain-relieving effects, however, which was to truly legitimize the procedure. One of the hottest subjects in contemporary neurochemistry is the endorphins. These are a family of peptides which have been found to be the body's natural opiates. Since it was discovered that narcotics such as morphine act by fooling brain receptors into thinking that they are the brain's own (i.e. endogenous) chemicals, the word endorphin is derived from 'endogenous morphine-like' substance.

The connection between endorphins and acupuncture was discovered by utilizing naloxone, a drug which prevents morphine from exerting its effects. Both human subjects and mice who showed evidence of relief from experimentally induced pain when given acupuncture failed to achieve pain relief when given naloxone prior to acupuncture (*Current Concepts in Pain and Analgesia* 4:8-9, 1977). More recently, endorphin levels in the cerebrospinal fluid which surrounds the brain have been shown to increase after acupuncture while areas in the brain which mediate pain and are rich in endorphins show a decline in their levels (*American Psychiatric Association News* 1 August 1980). As the final blow to the attempt to explain acupuncture as a form of hypnosis, it has recently been demonstrated that pain relief achieved through hypnosis is *not* blocked by naloxone; thus hypnosis, in contrast to acupuncture, is not mediated by endorphin release.

The establishment of a scientific basis for acupuncture which is consistent with western medical knowledge has made acupuncture respectable. Often forgotten, however, is the fact that acupuncture claims to be much more than merely a method of stimulating endorphin release. Its enthusiasts hold it to be a diagnostic method which can complement conventional diagnostic techniques as well as a treatment modality for a broad range of apparently unrelated illnesses.

To add to the complexity, each acupuncture point is believed to have specific effects when stimulated, effects which can vary according to such factors as the manner of stimulation, the nature of the illness, and even the time of day. There are several known microacupuncture systems which are believed to contain acupuncture points representing the entire body within a small area, of which the ear and foot systems are the most famous. There are also different methods of performing acupuncture; ear acupuncture, for example, can be practiced according to either the Chinese or the French method.

Research to attempt to validate the many facets of acupuncture has been sparse. So far, answers to only little pieces of the puzzle are emerging from scientific studies. For example, UCLA anesthesiologists have studied the accuracy of making a medical diagnosis by examining the acupuncture points in the ear. When forty patients with musculoskeletal pain were covered with sheets so that only their ears were exposed, the acupuncturist was able to establish the correct location for their pain through ear examination three-quarters of the time (Oleson *et al.*).

A major line of research has been to investigate the effects of stimulating specific acupuncture points. Effects have been described upon all the major systems of the body (Omura, O'Connor and Bensky). In order to avoid the effects of suggestion, the cardiovascular effects of needling certain acupuncture points has been studied on anesthetized dogs by anesthesiologists at the Medical College of Ohio (Lee *et al.*).

Unfortunately, most clinical studies of acupuncture are merely anecdotal case reports. While these reports are intriguing, and suggest a trial of acupuncture for many third line patients, they fail to establish whether acupuncture or other concurrent aspects of the treatment could be credited for the beneficial results.

We know that acupuncture *can* be effective, but we still know little about when it is best employed – other than from the recommendations of experienced clinicians. The New York State Commission on Acupuncture has reviewed the literature and suggests that the following conditions are frequently alleviated by or improved by acupuncture treatments (Riddle):

muscular spasms
  ex. tension headaches
    menstrual pain
    diarrhea
trigeminal neuralgia
hypertension
hypotension
chronic bronchitis
bronchial asthma
withdrawal symptoms in drug addicts
migraine headaches
arthritis (especially osteoarthritis)
insomnia
constipation
paralysis following strokes
functional disorders
post-herpetic neuralgia

There have been almost no studies comparing various treatment regimes using acupuncture. We do not know if one particular waveform emitted by a certain instrument which provides electrical stimulation of acupuncture points is more or less effective than any other waveform. We do not know if ear acupuncture is more or less effective than body acupuncture. We do not know if an experienced acupuncturist trained in the orient who uses needles and the concepts of traditional Chinese medicine (including pulse diagnosis and the Law of the Five Elements) obtains any better clinical results than a technician performing laser acupuncture with a 'cookbook' which prescribes a combination of points to stimulate for each condition being treated.

Nevertheless, we do know that acupuncture is often effective in a number of illnesses which have failed to respond to first and second line treatments. We also know that acupuncture is extremely safe, with few contraindications and minimal or no discomfort. That knowledge is enough to warrant a place for the procedure in Third Line Medicine.

CHAPTER 8
The third line approach

> The art of medicine . . . involves the ability to select, intuitively as it were, those aspects of the total medical situation in all its complexity which can be manipulated not only by scientific medical technologies but also by any other kind of influence which promises to be useful.
>
> RENÉ DUBOS
> 1901–82

The results are in. The weight of scientific evidence has disproven the doctrine of specific etiology which has dominated medical thought for the past century. Looking back, the doctrine was merely a fad in the course of medical history, a fad fueled by unbridled faith in the reductionist approach to illness which followed in the wake of Pasteur's germ theory. The new medicine has returned us to our roots in Hippocratean theory. The new physicians agree with the specific etiologists that specific agents are necessary for the development of certain diseases. Their model of illness, however, is systems-oriented and predicated upon their belief in the fundamental integrity of the bodymind.

Medical science is but one influence upon the practice of medicine, which is not a science, but an art which utilizes science. As an art, it is strongly influenced by its institutions, one of which is medical specialism which relegates the diagnosis and treatment of most serious illnesses to narrowly trained specialists who are ill equipped to deal with data which do not fit within the boundaries of their specialties. Specialization became necessary once the body of scientific knowledge became too vast for any one physician to be able to absorb it. Since this occurred during the height of popularity of the doctrine of specific etiology, specialties developed along lines which were consistent with the tenets of the doctrine. The development of psychiatry removed the responsibility of dealing with mental influences upon illness from the other areas of medical practice while it assumed only part of the burden itself. Other specialties developed which confined themselves to single organ systems or specific medical procedures, thus further tearing apart the human organism. The result was that subunits could be better examined, while the person who carried the illness became neglected.

The confirmation of ecologic theory by medical science has yet to become translated into major changes in the practice of medicine. This is because the medical establishment is built upon the tenets of specific etiology doctrine. The current system of medical education, for example, leaves little room for ecologic theory while it prepares medical students to choose their specialties. Each specialty has become a powerful interest group, with its own organization devoted to protecting its territorial rights. The practice of medicine desperately needs to be overhauled to better reflect ecologic concepts, but until this can be accomplished, I suggest that ecologic medicine can best be introduced into medical practice through the development of yet another specialty, a specialty I propose to call Third Line Medicine.

While Hippocrates is the father of ecologic medicine, John J. Bonica, Chief of Anesthesiology at the University of Washington in Seattle, was perhaps the first modern physician to champion a third line approach. Bonica, an anesthesiologist, has devoted his career to the treatment of pain syndromes. Pain is a symptom which crosses over the lines of most of the medical specialties. Prior to World War Two, each of these specialties had developed its own literature on the diagnosis and treatment of pain as it related to its own field, but no unified literature had developed on pain itself. Thus, when Bonica was called upon during World War Two to treat soldiers whose battle injuries had caused them to experience severe degrees of pain, he encountered two problems:

(a) research of the literature revealed that the available information was scattered through various journals; there

was no comprehensive source of information or reference work; and
(b) the use of traditional consultation by the specialists often failed to provide results. This prompted me to begin a systematic clinical study of various pain syndromes. . . . I also began to encourage neurosurgeons, orthopaedists, psychiatrists, and other colleagues to get together to discuss complex pain problems as a group. . . . This experience led me to the conclusion and development of the concept that in many instances correct diagnosis and effective therapy of difficult pain problems are possible only through the well coordinated and concerted efforts of the patient's doctor and a group of other specialists who contribute their individualized knowledge and skill for a common goal. (Bonica)

Immediately following the end of World War Two, Bonica began to preach his concept of a pain clinic. He directed one of the first pain clinics between 1947 and 1960 at Tacoma General Hospital; another was directed by F.A.D. Alexander at around the same time which was based on a similar concept (Alexander). In 1961, Bonica joined forces with a neurosurgeon, Lowell White, to found the pain clinic at the University of Washington which has served as a model for similar clinics throughout the world.

Directors of contemporary pain clinics are most often anesthesiologists, but neurologists, neurosurgeons, psychiatrists, psychologists, physiatrists, orthopedists and internists direct about one-third of them. The common modalities of treatment, in descending order of popularity, are nerve blocks, transcutaneous nerve stimulation, physical and occupational therapy, acupuncture, psychotherapy, behavior modification, biofeedback training and drug detoxification. One-third of the clinics employ a single physician; the rest utilize multiple specialists (*Stress/Pain Manager Newsletter* May, 1981).

The multi-disciplinary model of the pain clinic has demonstrated the value of extending the practice of medicine beyond the range of individual second line practitioners. It has also fostered research projects which, consonant with the ecologic model, investigate the multitude of factors which affect the genesis and maintenance of the symptom of pain. As a result, the experience of pain is now becoming recognized as being multidetermined; the reductionist labeling of pain as either 'real' (physical) or 'hysterical' (mental) has been clearly demonstrated to be inadequate.

Pain, of course, is not the only symptom which may fail to respond to Second Line Medicine. Recently, comprehensive behavioral medicine programs have become established in major medical centers which offer services to all patients who continue to be symptomatic after second line interventions. Behavioral medicine is defined as 'the *interdisciplinary* field concerned with the development and *integration* of behavioral and biomedical science, knowledge and techniques relevant to health and illness and the application of this knowledge and these techniques to prevention, diagnosis, treatment and rehabilitation.' (Schwartz and Weiss) According to Barry Blackwell of the University of Wisconsin Medical School, a behavioral medicine program is one which is 'designed to modify behavior (both gross illness behavior and discrete physiological behaviors) in people who have either evidence of (or a deep-seated conviction of) organic disease but who have failed to benefit from conventional biomedical treatments.' (Blackwell) For the program to be called comprehensive, Blackwell believes that an attempt must be made 'to evaluate each patient with regard to all the biological, social, and psychological variables before choosing the appropriate treatment(s).' (ibid.)

The multi-disciplinary pain center and the comprehensive behavioral medicine program are the first outposts of the new medicine accepted by the health care establishment. While the attempt to establish a specific diagnosis is not abandoned, the focus in these new fields is on applying techniques that work, whether or not the treatments are based upon the identification of a specific etiology for the presenting symptoms, and whether or not the mechanisms by which the treatments work are well understood. Each provides a limited form of Third Line Medicine – limited as regards to the pain center by the category of pain, and for the behavioral medicine program by its behavioral orientation. They are also limited by restricting themselves to procedures which are widely accepted in the medical community. Because of these limitations, many third line patients find that these programs have nothing to offer them.

The holistic health movement, on the other hand, is a recent innovation in medical care which has enthusiastically embraced controversial procedures. The movement, which burst upon the American scene in the mid-1970s, defines holistic health as: 'a state of well-being in which an individual's body, mind, emotions and spirit are in tune with the natural, cosmic and social environment.' (American Holistic Medical Association)

Holistic Medicine is defined as: 'a system of Health Care which emphasizes personal responsibility, and fosters a co-operative relationship among all those involved, leading toward optimal attunement of body, mind, emotions and spirit.' (ibid.)

The term 'holism' was first coined by the South African soldier and statesman Jan Smuts (1870–1950) who, in 1926, published a book titled *Holism and Evolution* in which he argued that evolution is a sequence of increasingly comprehensive integrations. Since then, others have extended Smuts' concept far beyond his original vision. Andras Angyal, for example, developed a holistic theory of personality. According to Angyal, personality 'is an organized whole and not a mere aggregate of discrete parts. Its functioning does not derive from the functioning of its parts; rather the parts must be viewed in the light of the organizational principles governing the whole.' (Angyal)

The extension of the concept of holism to the field of health is to be welcomed, since it returns the ancient ecologic principles of Hippocratic medicine to a position of legitimacy. In contrast to the medicine practiced by Hippocrates, and the concepts of holistic thinkers such as Smuts and Angyal, holistic health is primarily a grass roots movement which derives its popularity by providing an alternative to the form of medicine practiced by the specific etiologists whose influence dominates the medical establishment.

At least two independent trends have contributed to its growth and development. The first is the increasing disillusionment of the public with the current system of health care and its growing demand for an alternative manner of appraising states of health. One proposal for such an alternative which came to be adopted by the movement was made by Abraham Maslow (1908–70). Maslow believed that the rigid application of the scientific model of the physical sciences to psychology resulted in a fragmented picture of the human being, and urged the expansion of scientific study to include such vital areas as individuality and self-actualization. His emphasis on the study of healthy people who were seeking to fulfill their potentialities foreshadowed the movement's concern with 'optimal health' or 'high level wellness' as the alternative to the narrow disease-oriented model fostered by the specific etiologists.

The second trend which has strengthened the holistic health movement is the gradual erosion of the scientific and theoretical bases of the doctrine of specific etiology from within the medical establishment. Nowhere has this been more evident than at the forefront of medical research. As researchers in a number of highly specialized areas extend their investigations beyond their previous limits, they are discovering that, instead of diverging even further from the investigations of their colleagues, their work is increasingly intersecting. One result has been a gradual erosion of the mind-body split as newer, more integrated approaches combine both mental and physical elements in their protocols.

The new field of clinical biofeedback, for example, emerged a decade ago when experimental psychologists interested in behavior modification decided to attempt to apply the principles of operant conditioning to training the autonomic nervous system. Not only did they prove that this could be accomplished, but they also found that their work overlapped with the investigations of psychophysiologists (investigators concerned with the effects of mental processes upon the way the body functions) who were attempting to teach people how to exert voluntary control over the autonomic nervous system. Even more recent has been the development of the science of psychoimmunology which concerns itself with the influence of mental processes upon the immune system (Ader).

The return of ecologic medicine to a position of legitimacy within western medicine must certainly be fostered; there are reasons, however, to question whether the holistic health movement is the appropriate vehicle to represent it. While the basic concepts of holistic health are as wholesome as motherhood and apple pie, they are far too inclusive ever to be adequately defined in operational terms, and far too inclusive to be adequately critical of the vast fields it encompasses. An amalgam of popular fads and starry-eyed idealism combined with a pinch of science derived from the leading edge of medical research, the movement lacks any meaningful attempt at achieving an integration within itself. 'Holistic' is being used to describe any approach which deals with 'body, mind, emotions and spirit' as if it makes little difference how applicable, scientifically valid and cost-effective the approach may be. Patients entering the movement are greeted by a potpourri of diagnostic techniques and treatments to sample, often with little rationale for the items suggested for them to try. The emphasis is upon unvalidated procedures as if their rejection by the medical establishment somehow makes them better than conventional procedures.

Its anti-establishment posture, a legacy from the hippie movement, has gained the holistic health movement a great deal of popular support. Commercial firms have seen the value of utilizing the movement to increase the popularity of their products; the Holistic Products Corporation, for example, markets a Holistic Rectal Ointment which is fortified with bee propolis! The question is whether holistic health is really a forward move towards a more sophisticated, scientific and ecologic system of medical care or whether it is a step backward towards the era of patent medicines and other nostrums promoted for every illness a century ago.

Writing in the editorial column *The New England Journal of Medicine*, Arnold S. Relman has warned his readers that:

> It is important for us to recognize the limitations of medical technology in dealing with the human condition, and it is well to be reminded constantly . . . that patients must be dealt with as whole people. But this worthwhile philosophy is ill served by those who seek abandonment of science and rationality in favor of mystical cults. . . . A few years ago William G. Rothstein wrote an instructive history of *American Physicians in the Nineteenth Century*, which he subtitled 'From Sects to Science.' Let us hope that when the history of the holistic movement in medicine

> comes to be written it will not be entitled 'From Science to Sects.' (Relman)

Indeed, there is widespread concern among health care professionals over the manner in which the concept of holism is being translated into medical practice. Robert Ornstein, a psychologist at the University of California Medical Center, San Francisco and a leading authority on the study of consciousness, believes that:

> Holistic is a word that has become perverted. Holistic health is getting to be a fad. To many, it means only freaky things, so we end up with just another fragmented approach to health instead of a holistic one. Holistic is an attitude, not a system. Using chemotherapy to treat disease is not inconsistent with being holistic. The term should not be used to describe a system of treatment or an institute but an understanding of the whole situation. (Nelson)

Perhaps the problem with the holistic health movement lies in its grandiosity. Ecologic concepts are just beginning to seep into scientific research and the medical literature. Specialists speaking different professional languages are just starting to learn to translate between them, so that the same event can be described in, say, biochemical, neurophysiological or psychological terminology. However laudatory the concept may be, medical practice may not yet be ready for holism, even as a legitimate alternative to the established systems of front line and second line services. Until different lines of scientific research achieve further integrations, the amount of knowledge about each potentially contributory factor in illness may be too great for physicians to be able to master a truly holistic approach to general medical care.

Third Line Medicine, while rooted in the same ecologic model as holistic health, has much smaller, and thus more attainable aspirations. By restricting itself to patients who have already made the rounds of second line specialists, it does not attempt to include all of medicine within its bailiwick; instead it focuses on providing an integrated approach to the employment of those procedures which have either been neglected entirely, or have been utilized in a fragmented way which has mitigated their effectiveness. Only certain procedures are utilized – and only on certain people.

While aspects of Third Line Medicine are practiced by non-medical practitioners, third line physicians have the advantage of sharing a background in scientific medicine with their medical colleagues. In selecting their procedures, they review the available scientific evidence and give preference to the better validated procedures. As members of the same hospital staffs and medical societies, they speak the same language and share many of the same values with other physicians. These common bonds help assure continuity of care as the patient moves into Third Line Medicine. When this occurs, the transfer of medical responsibility is rarely complete, as first and second line physicians usually continue to provide primary care services.

Third Line Medicine also shares aspects of the approach favored by the other two lines of medical care. It shares with First Line Medicine a dedication to Hippocrates' ecologic model. With Second Line Medicine, it shares the devotion to exploring selected aspects of treatment in depth. As medical knowledge has expanded, other physicians can no longer maintain both broadness and depth without sacrificing the quality of their work. Third line physicians can do so only because the physicians who saw their patients previously have already performed numerous diagnostic and therapeutic procedures. The results of these procedures are already available, so that many of the issues which needed to be considered earlier are no longer relevant.

Third line physicians are not the exclusive providers of Third Line Medicine; it can also be provided by a team of second line practitioners. In this approach, exemplified by the multi-disciplinary pain clinic, patients are evaluated and treated by various team members. Coordination is provided by regular staff conferences and the assignment of patient managers. Input provided by individual team members helps correct for the distortions in perspective usually encountered in Second Line Medicine without sacrificing the depth of knowledge which second line physicians have acquired. Not all of the members of the team need be physicians; indeed, even the team director does not have to be a physician so long as adequate medical expertise is provided by the team.

Since third line patients are defined by their failure to respond to second line procedures, they may appear to constitute a very heterogeneous group. In fact, they have much in common. They do not require routine medical examinations, since these examinations have already been performed, usually several times, by previous physicians, and will continue to be performed by the physicians responsible for their primary care. They often complain of symptoms which are common to many disorders (pain, fatigue and malaise are examples) or present with a catalog of complaints.

In addition, third line patients display the psychological characteristics which develop when illness becomes chronic (Abram). Their symptoms have gradually eroded their capacity to accept them. Depression is usually present, even though it may be hidden or denied, as is anger born of frustration. They are caught between hope and despair. Hope has brought them to Third Line Medicine, but they are on the verge of sinking into the abyss of despair.

We can readily group third line patients into three categories. People in the first category have physical complaints with demonstrable structural or chemical abnormalities which seem to explain their discomfort. Third line practitioners see patients in this group whose symptoms have failed to respond adequately to appropriate medical and surgical interventions. Examples would be people with symptoms following bodily injury and people with degenerative diseases.

The second category consists of people whose physical findings are not adequate to account for the severity of their symptoms; thus their physicians will commonly consider these 'excessive' symptoms to be entirely psychological in origin. In order to reach the doorway to Third Line Medicine, they have either refused formal psychiatric treatment, or have already seen second line psychiatrists but remain ill even after lengthy treatment attempts.

The third category consists of people with physical complaints found to be due to changes in the way their bodies function. Examples are patients with spastic colitis, muscle contraction or vascular headaches, and tachycardia (rapid heart beat). Since they return frequently to their doctors for changes and renewals of medications over a long period of time, they constitute a substantial percentage of many physicians' practices. Usually, the members of this group who reach third line physicians are those who either have not responded to second line treatments, or who have sought Third Line Medicine on their own.

What can Third Line Medicine offer these patients which is not available from Second Line Medicine? The answer lies in the reductionist approach, based on the doctrine of specific etiology, which underlies the practice of Second Line Medicine. Second line physicians generally limit their investigations to procedures which keep them safely within the confines of their respective specialties. They first screen the clinical problem through a grid which selects out the features of the case which are most pertinent to their area of specialization. The information base within the grid is then expanded by means of further evaluative procedures which fall within the limits of their speciality; at the same time, data which do not fit within the grid are excluded.

Let us suppose that the patient is a man with persistent headaches. As part of their evaluation, an orthopedist might order x-rays of the cervical spine, a neurologist might order an electroencephalogram, an allergist might perform scratch testing, and a psychiatrist might order psychological testing. If any of their respective procedures produce positive findings, those findings will suggest a diagnosis which fits within that specialty. Treatment will then be predicated upon that diagnosis and will consist of procedures known to be effective for symptoms produced by that illness.

When the factors contributing to the genesis and maintenance of the symptom are multiple, or when these factors are not discovered by routine diagnostic testing, second line procedures are likely to fail. Viable treatment options remain, but these are often avoided by second line physicians as they do not fit within the limits of their specialties. These procedures are derived from the ecologic model and are not specific to the treatment of any one disease. Instead, they seek to intercede with mechanisms of symptom production which are common to many disease states.

Another reason why second line physicians may fail to help patients who could benefit from Third Line Medicine is their avoidance of controversial procedures. Procedures are generally considered to be controversial so long as the bulk of practitioners do not approve of their use in clinical practice while a smaller group disagrees and employs them. Usually the criticism of these procedures is based on the claim of the larger group that there is insufficient scientific evidence of their efficacy to warrant their introduction.

In Chapter Four we reviewed the nature of modern scientific information. We saw how research contributes to medical knowledge, but is inadequate as the sole basis for making clinical decisions. Immanuel Kant (1724–1804), one of the greatest philosophers of all time, has suggested that: 'It is often necessary to make decisions on the basis of knowledge which is sufficient for action but insufficient to satisfy the intellect.'

Procedures which the experts believe to have achieved adequate scientific validation for their introduction into clinical medicine are those which satisfy the intellect of most clinicians. These procedures, however, have already been found to be ineffective for patients who reach third line physicians. They are a unique group of people who deserve a chance to respond to clinical interventions which are based on lower levels of information.

C. Norman Shealy, a prominent neurosurgeon, asserts that:

> the quality of medical and health care can be improved by . . . allowing a genuine difference of philosophy to persist when there is no 'proven' effectiveness. Surely any treatment which is logically safe and which has been empirically demonstrated to be reasonably safe is acceptable . . . *as long as it does not prevent the patient from receiving a truly lifesaving, scientifically documented, effective treatment.* (Shealy)

Safe but poorly validated treatments have been accused by their detractors of being riddled with placebo effects. They are correct, of course, but if a treatment is effective for a third line patient, what difference does it make whether a placebo effect was responsible for the patient's improvement? In fact, much of the effectiveness of validated treatments in clinical settings can also be traced to their placebo components, as scientific studies do no more than prove that the experimental treatments were at least slightly more effective in the experimental setting than the particular type of placebo employed in the study.

On the other hand, controversial procedures should only be introduced into the practice of Third Line Medicine under certain conditions. Physicians must first become knowledgeable about *both* sides of the controversy and must present the nature of the controversy to their patients in an objective and balanced manner so that they can have a rational basis for deciding if they wish to try the procedure. Procedures should only be introduced for a specific trial period and then withdrawn to see if symptoms return in the event that there is doubt concerning their effectiveness. Only procedures which appear to be particularly safe and devoid of adverse side effects should be suggested.

Finally, when presenting controversial procedures to their patients, third line physicians should give preference to procedures which they have personally employed long enough to reach their own conclusions as to their efficacy. There are two reasons for this. This first is because an author's advocacy of a controversial procedure is particularly subject to that person's biases. The other is that, since trials of the procedure have been limited, differences between the patients on whom the procedure was reported and the patients being seen by the third line physician may be great enough to affect the results.

Yet another reason why first and second line practitioners may have failed to satisfy their patients' needs for symptom relief lies in the manner in which they dealt with, or failed to deal with, psychological issues. In a medical world dominated by specific etiologists, pity the poor people who experience physical distress when no structural or chemical abnormalities can be found to 'justify' the severity of their symptoms. These sufferers are the second-class citizens of the medical world; their physicians eye them with suspicion as they feel that these patients have tried to fool them into believing that they have 'real' illnesses.

Physicians who believe that the lack of an identified disease process makes an illness less real will in subtle, and sometimes not so subtle, ways distance themselves from these patients. Instead of investigating physiological and biochemical influences upon their symptoms, they will quickly turn to prescribing tranquilizers and antidepressants. The most notorious example has been the overprescription of Valium (c), a tranquilizer which has become the most widely prescribed medication in America, and the most economically successful medication in the history of the world. While an excellent muscle relaxant as well as an effective tranquilizer, the misuse of Valium (c) can lead either to a pattern of increasing drug dependency or a worsening of depression.

More fortunate are those patients who are referred to psychiatrists, since they are devoted to helping people who have been labeled as mentally ill – even though psychiatrists, like other second line physicians, are prone to blame disorders with no apparent structural causes on psychopathology. Many of these patients will never arrive at the psychiatrists' offices, however. Since they share the same biases as their physicians, they may view a psychiatric referral as an accusation that they are not really ill and may refuse to accept a psychiatric label. This may explain why psychosomatic patients have been found to evidence a considerably lower degree of motivation for psychiatric treatment than neurotic patients and are more defensive in their attitudes toward what the psychiatrist believes to be their mental problems (Salminen *et al.*).

While much has been written concerning the psychiatric treatment of psychosomatic disorders, its effectiveness is uncertain. There is a lack of well-designed, controlled studies investigating the efficacy of psychotherapy in this area (Kellner), although it does appear that 'treatment is generally a long-term proposition.' (Stevens) Similarly, most of the applications of behavior therapy to psychosomatic disorders have not been experimentally investigated (Price). Suffice it to say that many of the patients referred to psychiatrists because of physical symptoms which have no apparent structural cause, will fail to benefit from the referral.

Most third line patients do have significant psychological problems. Some of these problems, especially regarding feelings of anger, fear and depression, will have been fueled by the persistence of their symptoms. Others, such as a need to manipulate others through the use of their symptoms, may not only have etiologic relevance, but may prevent symptom resolution until they have been resolved. There are also some patients who have remarkable psychological strength which has sustained them through a most stressful period in their lives. These patients are a delight for third line practitioners, as they present neither conscious nor unconscious resistance to the efficacy of third line techniques and frequently make a smooth and rapid recovery once an appropriate treatment is initiated.

Third line physicians have a distinct advantage over their second line psychiatric colleagues when dealing with psychological issues. Since a referral to a third line physician does not label the patient as 'psychiatric', third line practitioners evaluate and treat many patients who would not be willing to be formally seen by psychiatrists. They share with second line psychiatrists, however, an understanding of the psychological aspects of illness, an understanding which influences their evaluations, treatments and interactions with their patients. They analyze the dynamic interactions between patients and staff for clues to hidden psychological issues which can influence the course of their illnesses. Psychoanalytic concepts such as transference, resistance and ego defenses are well understood and utilized as are the concepts of behavior modification.

While most physicians now recognize the deleterious effects of such personal behaviors as smoking, drinking, overworking and lack of exercise, third line physicians go beyond merely prescribing behavioral changes. They recognize that, even though patients may have physical diseases, harmful personal behaviors which may instigate the diseases are often the result of underlying psychological issues. If so, the behaviors will most likely continue until those issues are dealt with adequately.

They seek to minimize the authoritarian aspects of the doctor-patient relationship as well as any differences between doctor and patient concerning treatment goals. Patients are encouraged to share in the formulation of the treatment plan and are educated so that they can participate in discussions in a meaningful and productive way. When they are reluctant to endorse a proposed plan of treatment, third line physicians will suggest an alternative plan which better fits their wishes. Active collaborators rather than passive recipients of the doctor's wisdom, third line patients who previously failed to comply with their doctors' orders often form a healing partnership with third line physicians.

All interactions between patients and staff are analyzed and dealt with from the sophisticated perspective of the psychotherapist. The way the secretaries deal with patients on the telephone is considered as relevant as a formal psychotherapy session, both for gaining an understanding of the patients' psyches and for intervening in ways which are potentially therapeutic. The entire staff, both secretarial and professional, meets regularly to discuss issues which involve their relationships with their patients in order to better understand and interact with them. Even interactions between staff members concerning patients are discussed, as patients may unconsciously seek to recreate their familial relationships within the office setting by fostering alliances or splits among staff.

There are certain differences between this informal psychotherapeutic milieu and formal psychotherapy. Patients are never confronted about inappropriate behavior except by the professionals with whom they are actively involved in treatment. Even then, confrontation is only done when patients seem receptive to receiving it. While the atmosphere is one which facilitates communication of feelings and the professional staff encourages patients to share information about their personal lives, patients are never pressured to reveal any more personal material than they wish to share. Finally, psychotherapeutic issues are considered to be only supplementary to the formal agenda for the sessions unless both patient and professional decide to make them primary.

Patients who refuse or resist formal psychotherapy often begin to open up and share their inner thoughts and feelings in the informal psychotherapeutic milieu. This is particularly true when relaxation training techniques are part of their treatment program, since people feel less threatened about self-exposure as they learn to relax. Once they have begun to recognize that it is safe and even beneficial to look inwards, patients who previously had been resistent to the idea of psychotherapy despite their evident need for it become more accepting of the procedure.

American psychiatry is currently divided into three major schools, the psychoanalytic, the behavioral and the biological, and subdivided into dozens of camps. Each camp claims superiority over its rivals while, in fact, each concentrates its treatment efforts upon the sector of the psychiatric population for which its methods are most effective. This arrangement works well for patients who are only appropriate for one form of treatment. When, however, patients are appropriate candidates for various treatments, the choice of treatment is likely to be more dependent upon the choice of psychiatrist than upon the relative merits of the procedures.

Fortunately, an increasing number of psychiatrists have recognized the inadequacy of this situation. These new psychiatrists, like other practitioners of the new medicine, have gone back to their Hippocratean roots to embrace a model derived from general systems theory (Meir). Their approach is called 'eclectic' which, according to *Webster's New Collegiate Dictionary*, means 'selecting what appears to be best in various doctrines, methods, or styles.' Writing in the *Archives of General Psychiatry*, Gene Abroms, a strong advocate of psychiatric eclecticism, states that:

> The meaningful struggle in our field now is not between simplistic explanatory slogans but whether we are going to continue to train therapists, as in the past, to use only one or two treatment techniques which apply to an elite group of patients, or instead to make them masters of a large repertoire of methods capable of helping those who at one time never came or were forced to 'drop out.' (Abroms)

Unlike the advocates of holistic health, eclectic psychiatrists have struggled with the failure of general systems theory to provide guidelines for the rational selection of treatments. Robert M. Simon, writing in the *American Journal of Psychiatry*, suggests that:

> we might call eclectic choices artistic ones. . . . Such choices are impervious to scientific understanding at the present, and it may be that what we now know as art and science will have to be integrated before the issue of eclecticism . . . is finally resolved. In the meantime it continues to attract practitioners but to run the risk of resulting in dilettantism and therefore the risk of being rejected by the profession. (Simon)

Third line physicians share the same basic model, and thus are susceptible to the same risks, as eclectic psychiatrists. They are well grounded in the art of medicine, but unless they follow certain guidelines in their protocols, they are in danger of wandering too far from the bastion of science. They should give preference, for example, to procedures which have some scientific validation over otherwise equivalent procedures which have none. Procedures which have been proven ineffective should be avoided. If a firm diagnosis has not been established, they should give preference to procedures which can establish one. Each treatment should be recommended only for a specific, limited period of time; if the patient has not received significant benefits by the end of that time, the treatment should be abandoned.

Other factors should also influence their choice of procedures. They must be acutely aware of non-specific (placebo) effects and attempt to harness those effects in a manner which maximizes the patient's chance for improvement. For example, they should give preference to procedures for which patients have positive expectations, since expectancy can influence outcome. The relative cost of each procedure should be weighed, as should the physical and emotional discomfort each would entail.

In contrast to the other medical specialties, Third Line Medicine does not focus its assessment procedures upon the establishment of a definitive diagnosis. Third line patients have already been subjected to numerous diagnostic procedures which are likely to have led to the establishment of a diagnosis so long as the illness is one which can be classified. Second line physicians are the expert diagnosticians; if they could not reach a diagnosis, it is unlikely that third line physicians will be able to do so. Besides, diagnosis, while useful, is closely tied with the simplistic notions of the doctrine of specific etiology. By pointing the finger at a single cause for the illness, a diagnosis tends to encourage physicians to neglect to attend to the other causative factors.

In other words, Third Line Medicine stresses the general assessment of the patient's condition and the factors which both initiated and maintain the state of illness, while de-emphasizing specific diagnoses. Assessment is seen as an ongoing process, for each bit of new information gained from contact with patients as they proceed through a treatment program modifies earlier impressions and recommendations.

There is also a de-emphasis on physical examinations as compared to First and Second Line Medicine. Third line patients have had repeated physicals by well-trained physicians; by the time they reach third line physicians, it is highly unlikely that new physical findings will be discovered. In addition, patients' primary physicians continue to follow them while they are receiving third line care so that changes in physical findings will not be missed.

There is a place, however, for a physical exam. The experiential contact between physician and patient which is made when the doctor feels an area of the body in which the patient experiences distress does something for both parties. The physician becomes more appreciative of the physical aspects of the patient's condition, while the patient feels better understood.

Third line physicians presume that mental processes are involved in all illnesses and have etiologic relevance at multiple points in both their genesis and maintenance. They seek to discover what their patients' symptoms mean to them on both conscious and unconscious levels. They wonder, for example, if illness is scorned or fearfully pampered by their nuclear family. Do family members control others through illness or use illness as an excuse to avoid taking responsibility for their actions? What specific illnesses has the family had to deal with, how did it deal with them, and did those illnesses resolve?

They review the situational factors which existed just prior to the onset of the illness. Had the person been stressed by recent life events? Was he or she in a relationship which was becoming intolerable but which couldn't be avoided? What rewards, if any, could illness bring at that time? Once the illness started how did it change the person's life? Did angry relatives ask forgiveness? Is the boss finally off the person's back? Has the fear, pain or anger generated by the disability begun to interfere with the person's desire to recover?

They also review the events which transpired after the illness became manifest in order to assess their influence upon the clinical course. When health professionals entered the picture, for example, how did they relate to the patient? Were they compassionate or distant, caring or uninterested? Did they blame the patient for not responding to their ministrations or did they provide ongoing support and encouragement? To third line practitioners, all these issues may be affecting the course of the illness. When they are found to be influential, they must be dealt with in order to improve the chances for recovery.

Concern for the patient's general sense of well-being permeates all third line procedures. Regardless of their efficacy in alleviating the presenting symptoms, these procedures may result in a number of beneficial non-specific effects. These effects, such as improved mood, improved self-control, personal insights or greater energy, can be so powerful that patients often feel satisfied with their treatments even when the treatments have failed to alleviate their presenting symptoms.

Treatments in Third Line Medicine are primarily directed at strengthening the organism's own adaptive mechanisms. This approach contrasts with most first and second line procedures which attempt to impose arbitrary biological changes through external means. The latter treatments are more dangerous as the changes they impose operate independently of the organism's ability to adapt to them. In other words, the effects of interventions which reinforce the organism's inherent capabilities are modulated by biological feedback mechanisms which protect the organism from changes which exceed its capacity to adapt to them. Treatments such as drugs and surgery lack the protection offered by these mechanisms as changes are imposed without regard for the organism's adaptive capabilities.

The issue of safety is important in regard to all treatments, but never more so than in Third Line Medicine, since third line patients already bear the scars from previous treatments, scars which make them reluctant to risk further adverse effects. Because of their safety, third line treatments are often assumed to be less effective. This is an unfortunate assumption which is not borne out, since third line procedures can be strikingly effective even after the more 'heroic' procedures have failed.

Procedures which are available in Second Line Medicine are offered, when indicated, but only if the patient's other treating physicians do not offer them or request third line physicians to provide them in order to better coordinate treatment services while the patient remains under third line care. Thus standard psychiatric procedures, such as psychological testing, psychotherapy and hypnotherapy may be provided. Third line physicians will usually assume responsibility for prescribing addicting medications. If they wish to make other changes in medications, they will discuss these proposals with the other treating physicians and defer to their decisions.

Third Line Medicine is limited to utilizing procedures which share the following four characteristics:

1 They are not commonly utilized by first and second line physicians.
2 They work by strengthening natural adaptive mechanisms.
3 They are relatively safe.
4 They are relatively non-specific; i.e. variations of one procedure are applicable to many different clinical problems and the beneficial effects of the procedure are not limited to its effects upon the presenting symptoms.

The specific content of third line practice is fluid. As time passes, some third line procedures will slowly permeate into the rest of medical practice because of increasing popularity due, perhaps, to more definitive scientific validation. Other third line procedures will be discarded as they have failed to live up to expectations. Newer procedures will replace those which are abandoned. Many of these will emerge from the vast caldron of folk medicine as the results of early studies provide some evidence of their efficacy, while others will develop directly out of office practice as clinical trials prove them to be effective.

It is obvious that third line physicians should have an unusually broad medical background. Fundamental must be a thorough knowledge of the relationship of mental processes to illness. Psychiatry, as a second line specialty, has developed the major portion of this body of knowledge, particularly in the emerging sub-specialty of liaison psychiatry which attempts to bridge some of the gap between physicians with somatic and those with psychological orientations (Lipowski). Related areas, such as learning theory, psychophysiology and psychoimmunology must also be included in their curriculum.

Some knowledge of the second line specialties, especially internal medicine, neurology, endocrinology and allergy, must be gained. Knowledge of clinical nutrition is imperative as is an appreciation of the history and general principles upon which the ecologic approach is based. Controversial procedures which appear to be of clinical utility must be studied in depth so that practitioners can reach their own conclusions as to their applicability. If they are to avoid the twin pitfalls of pseudoscience and dogma, a thorough understanding of the scientific method and medical statistics is vital.

The practice of Third Line Medicine thus requires an extensive educational background which builds upon basic medical training in a manner analagous to other forms of specialty care. Until residencies are established for physicians wishing to pursue this field, third line practitioners must come from the traditional specialties and seek to expand their horizons without the benefits of formalized training programs. The extensive post-residency training that is involved, and the lack of well-delineated guidelines for such training, has so far restricted the population of competent third line practitioners to a small number of physicians. Their number appears to be growing although, since there is yet to be a formal means of identifying them, nobody knows how many physicians actually practice at least some aspects of Third Line Medicine as defined herein. In any case, there are two reasons why Third Line Medicine should gradually emerge as an essential component of our system of contemporary medical practice. First, the third line approach is increasingly being validated by medical science, and second, patients will be pleased with the benefits it provides them.

CHAPTER 9
Cures for nondisease

Apollo, great and good clinician
Make me an able *non*clinician.
Teach me how to recognize
A *non*disease in *non*disguise.

GEORGE M. BRENIER
The New England Journal of Medicine
25 February 1965

Medicine, according to *Stedman's Medical Dictionary*, is 'the art of preventing or curing disease; the science that treats disease in all its relations.' Disease, the dictionary tells us, is characterized by at least two of the following criteria:

1 A recognized etiologic agent (or agents)
2 An identifiable group of signs and symptoms
3 Consistent anatomical alterations

We can conclude from these definitions that practicing physicians are trained to deal with those patients who are found, upon evaluation, to qualify as suffering from a disease. But what about the many patients who seek medical attention for their symptoms but no disease can be identified?

These sufferers have been evaluated by their first line physicians and no objective findings were apparent. Because of their distress, they were referred to second line physicians for more detailed evaluations, but once again no objective findings were noted. Usually, at this point, their complaints were labeled as psychogenic and treated as if a psychological cause had been proven. Treatment would include reassurance, the prescription of anti-anxiety medications, or referral to a psychiatrist.

Clifton Meador, a faculty member of the University of Alabama Medical Center, has suggested (perhaps with tongue in cheek) a method of classifying the medical diagnosis of these patients. Since they are sent to specific second line physicians because their signs and symptoms resemble those of a recognized disease yet, upon evaluation, they are found to not have that disease, Meador proposes that they be diagnosed as having a 'nondisease.' The problem, notes Meador, is that 'patients when told of their overt nondisease tend to become hostile and difficult to manage. Nonanxiety becomes anxiety.' (Meador)

This assumption, that the failure to diagnose a disease proves that the patient is suffering from a nondisease, is often tragic in its effects. Many of these people do have nondisease; in many cases, the origin of their complaints is in their psyches rather than in their somas. However, many others who have been dismissed by second line physicians as being afflicted by nondisease have real diseases which their physicians are poorly equipped to diagnose.

There are good reasons for their failure to recognize the diagnosis. First of all, these patients fail to display any 'consistent anatomical alterations'. Second line physicians are well equipped to discover structural abnormalities of the body, but attempts to find pathology in these patients will be futile. Second, the agents responsible for their diseases do not fit within any of the definitions of the areas of interest of the established medical specialties. Finally, the physical and behavioral signs and symptoms of these diseases often fail to be specific enough to be diagnostic of any one disease.

MARGINAL VITAMIN DEFICIENCY

Marginal vitamin deficiency is an excellent example of the type of diagnosis missed by second line specialists. Gross vitamin deficiencies like scurvy, beriberi and pellagra are quite rare today and are relatively easy to diagnose. Is there a grey area between adequate cellular levels of vitamins and frank deficiencies which may produce some of the symptoms of vitamin deficiencies but not the full picture needed for diagnosis?

The answer is a definite yes. Marginal vitamin deficiencies

have been identified and have been found to produce a variety of non-specific symptoms including:

fatigue
lack of appetite
depression
irritability
headaches
palpitations
difficulty concentrating
aches and pains

These symptoms have been produced in humans given vitamin deficient diets who showed no physical signs of vitamin deficiencies. When the vitamins lacking in their diet were replaced, the symptoms abated (Brozek, Hodges *et al.*, Sterner and Price).

All the above symptoms could be due to changes in brain function creating depression and anxiety which, in turn, could be partially expressed by physical complaints. Other studies have shown, however, that marginal vitamin deficiencies also have pronounced effects on other systems of the body. The metabolism of both drugs and environmental chemicals, for example, has been shown to be markedly affected by such marginal deficiencies (Brin, 1978). Similarly, marginal vitamin deficiencies have been shown to result in significant impairment of the immune system (Axelrod).

In contrast to gross vitamin deficiencies, marginal deficiencies are not uncommon. Recently, it has become possible to detect marginal deficiencies by the use of sensitive assay procedures which measure the activity of enzymes within the red blood cells. Since the activity of these enzymes depends upon adequate supplies of the proper vitamins, marginal deficiencies will be reflected by diminished enzyme activity even when serum levels of the vitamin are normal.

Thiamine nutriture, for example, can be most accurately assessed by measuring red blood cell transketolase (Massod *et al.*). Lonsdale and Shamberger have demonstrated that patients who complain of physical and emotional symptoms which appear to be neurotic in origin may actually be suffering from a marginal deficiency of this important B vitamin. Some of the many symptoms described by a group of twenty patients who were found to have abnormal transketolase activity were:

Chest and/or abdominal pains (with no physical findings)
Sleep disturbances
Personality changes
Recurrent fevers (of unknown origin)
Diarrhea
Chronic fatigue
Excessive sweating (usually at night)

According to the authors:

> The symptoms in our patients were those considered generally to be those of neurotic dysfunction, conversion reactions or hysterical conditions that are frequently treated by sedatives and psychological counsel.

None of the patients demonstrated the classical signs and symptoms of beriberi, the thiamine deficiency disease. After supplementation with thiamine, however, both transketolase activity and their sense of well-being improved (Lonsdale and Shamberger).

Myron Brin explains such results by postulating five stages in the development of a vitamin deficiency. In the preliminary stage, there is reduction of the tissue stores of the vitamin and depression of its excretion in the urine. Next, in the biochemical stage, enzymes requiring the vitamin begin to demonstrate reduced activity. In stage three, the physiological, behavioral effects such as insomnia or somnolence, irritability, and loss of appetite become apparent. These effects can be measured but are not specific to any particular deficiency.

Stage four is the clinical stage. This is the stage in which the classical vitamin deficiency disease syndrome develops, and the stage upon which the RDAs are based. The fifth stage is the terminal stage. In this stage, there will be severe tissue damage which, in the continued absence of the vitamin, will result in death.

Brin notes that the first three stages can be described as marginal vitamin deficiency and has presented research findings which are consistent with his model (Brin, 1979 and 1980). The implication is that marginal vitamin deficiencies may not only exist among people ingesting the recommended dietary allowances, but that these deficiencies may produce serious but non-specific physical and mental symptoms in the absence of any evidence of a classical vitamin deficiency disease.

Rather than pooling subjects on the basis of one specific deficiency, Laraine Abbey has reported on a group of patients with one specific illness: agoraphobia. This illness, which literally means a fear of open places, is better described as a fear of leaving a place of safety. It begins with one or more acute and inexplicable attacks of panic with such symptoms as palpitations, breathing difficulties, dizziness and sweatiness. Soon, patients become fearful that going away from their 'safe place' will result in another attack. They begin to avoid activities and gradually confine themselves more and more to their home, to staying with a trusted person, or otherwise keeping within their safe zone.

While agoraphobia is considered to belong within the province of psychiatry, the results of psychotherapy have been uniformly poor, and only recently has there been some evidence that certain psychotropic drugs may be of value (Zitrin *et al.*). Abbey performed functional vitamin assays for six of the B vitamins on twelve out of a group of twenty-three agoraphobics. *All* were found to have one or more marginal deficiencies. The entire group was given megadoses of nutrients and, three months later, nineteen of the twenty-three had dramatic improvements in their condition (Abbey).

ESSENTIAL FATTY ACID DEFICIENCIES

Donald Rudin has done some interesting work which suggests that some people may require larger than normal intakes of the B vitamins or may even fail to respond to megadoses because of another nutritional deficiency, namely a deficiency of a particular group of fatty acids in the modern diet. These fatty acids (the omega 3 family) are normally converted, in the presence of the proper vitamins and other factors, into prostaglandins – hormones with powerful effects upon brain function as well as upon all the tissues of the body. When they are deficient, prostaglandin deficiencies will also develop.

Megadoses of the B vitamins may help to push the conversion of fatty acids into prostaglandins but, in this case, they are not the cause of the problem and thus cannot solve it (Rudin 1982 and 1983).

Rudin has described a group of twelve patients with schizophrenia, manic depressive illness or agoraphobia as well as a number of other medical problems, notably:

skin lesions (especially drying dermatoses)
fatigue
autonomic dysfunctions (cold intolerance, bowel complaints, etc.)
tinnitus (i.e. ringing in the ears)
food sensitivities
osteoarthritis
menstrual irregularities
alcohol intolerance

Patients were treated with carefully titrated doses of linseed oil, an oil high in omega 3 essential fatty acids. Within one or two weeks, all eight patients with relapsing symptoms began to improve. Within six to eight weeks, improvement was usually marked in regard to all of their symptoms. Only the four patients whose symptoms were fixed (i.e. did not wax and wane) failed to improve (Rudin 1981).

David Horrobin, formerly a professor at Oxford University and the University of Montreal, is an internationally recognized authority on the prostaglandins. He has suggested on the basis of both direct and indirect evidence that a number of different diseases and syndromes ranging from schizophrenia and hyperactivity to multiple sclerosis, allergy and diabetes may be facilitated by a deficiency of prostaglandin E 1, normally derived from the omega 6 essential fatty acids. If so, evening primrose oil, an oil with the highest amount of the proper prostaglandin precursor outside of human breast milk, may be of benefit (Horrobin).

Currently, over a hundred clinical trials of evening primrose oil are underway or have been recently completed in thirteen countries. Early results are suggesting that it may be beneficial in:

lowering blood pressure
reducing risk of thrombosis (blood clots)
lowering serum cholesterol
relieving hangovers
improving behavior in hyperactive children
relieving premenstrual syndrome
alleviating breast pain
treating eczema
treating brittle nails
attenuating schizophrenic symptoms ('Efamol' technical information bulletins)

While more double-blind studies need to be done before we know how beneficial it may be to attempt to manipulate fatty acid levels, the results of a number of studies are suggesting that fatty acid abnormalities are one of the factors responsible for a wide range of conditions – some of which are still being considered non-diseases by most clinicians.

HEAVY METAL TOXICITY

Just as in the case of nutritional deficiencies, certain heavy metals can exert a toxic effect upon the various body tissues to produce a wide array of signs and symptoms. When industrial workers develop peculiar symptoms, the possibility of them having been exposed to a toxic substance is usually investigated. Few physicians, however, would even think that heavy metals placed permanently within the mouth by dentists could be the source of the illness, yet the evidence is growing that dental fillings and restorations are responsible for the development of significant illness in some people.

Mercury is generally acknowledged to be one of the most toxic of all metals, yet a sizeable portion of the population has had mercury permanently installed in their teeth as a component of their silver amalgam fillings. Organized dentistry has insisted that silver amalgams are safe, but are they? Let us review the evidence.

Following the placement of silver amalgams, measurable levels of mercury are expired with each breath (Gay *et al.*). The maximum permissible level of exposure to mercury vapor in industry (i.e. 40 hours of exposure out of the 168 hours in a week) is 50 micrograms per cubic meter and will soon be lowered to 25 micrograms (Hursch *et al.*). Fertile women should not be exposed to vapor levels above 10 micrograms and pregnant women not to any raised levels at all since mercury rapidly passes over to the fetus (Koos and Longo). Symptoms suggestive of mercury poisoning have been reported at levels below 3 micrograms (Stock, 1939). Because Soviet studies have shown biological effects at even a few micrograms (Trachtenberg), the USSR has established a safe limit for continuous mercury exposure in living quarters at 0.3 micrograms (Hanson).

The level of mercury vapor in expired air from people who have silver amalgam fillings has been studied for half a century. The results of these studies, reviewed in the light of the above data, are hardly reassuring. Most recently, for example, a study published in *Lancet* found baseline levels of 2.8 micrograms which increased to 49 micrograms when the subjects chewed gum (Gay *et al.*). Values of up to 87.5 micrograms were reported in a study published in the *Journal of Dental Research* which also found that the levels were proportional to the number of fillings (Svare *et al.*).

As the years pass, the dangers of mercury poisoning may well increase because of the gradual corrosion of the amalgam which will release mercury into the surrounding tissues (Hanson). The rate of corrosion is significantly increased when an amalgam is placed adjacent to an older amalgam, an amalgam of different composition, or gold (ibid.). This is due to the fact that a galvanic (electrical) cell is created (Pelva).

Chronic mercury poisoning can sometimes be diagnosed by assaying mercury levels in the blood, hair or urine. Unfortunately, these levels may be entirely normal despite the presence of advanced symptoms, although they may fall dramatically as soon as the last amalgam is removed (Hanson). There is one laboratory study, the white blood cell count, which is frequently at least mildly elevated in affected people, and that finding (WBC over 11,000 for three months without visible medical cause), along with a suspicious clinical picture, has been suggested as a criterion for deciding upon the removal of all amalgams (ibid.).

The picture of chronic mercury poisoning, just as the picture of the other diseases described in this chapter, is quite varied and involves multiple organ systems. Three features are relatively common. The first, *stomatitis*, refers to inflammation of the lining of the mouth and gums. Early symptoms may be tenderness or ready bleeding of the gums upon brushing. Frequent complaints are of excessive salivation or a metallic taste. The second is *neuromuscular* symptoms, such as tremors, jerky movements and deteriorating coordination, as well as increasing fatigue.

The last is *erethism*, a psychic disturbance of insidious onset. This may be the most prominent feature, and may lead to a prolonged course of inappropriate psychiatric treatment. Those afflicted become increasingly shy, nervous and irritable. As time goes on, they begin to withdraw from friends and family and become increasingly depressed.

The good news is that, as soon as the last amalgam is removed, there is a rapid recovery. Alfred Stock, a professor of biochemistry, published a paper in 1926 documenting his suffering from mercury toxicity due to dental amalgams until he made his own diagnosis and had the amalgams removed (Stock 1926). Afterwards he conducted a series of research studies which laid the groundwork for our current knowledge in this area. More recently, Jaro Pleva, a researcher in the field of metal corrosion, was similarly afflicted and, in the tradition of Stock, diagnosed his own condition after giving up on finding the answer from the medical profession and then proceeded to apply his expertise to advancing our knowledge (Pleva).

It should also be noted that the electrical potentials resulting from amalgams appear to be large enough to cause symptoms by themselves, so that the dissolution of mercury may not be necessary to explain the development of illness. Headaches, facial pains, dizziness, nausea, ringing in the ears and psychological disorders are some of the symptoms which have been reported to be associated with increased electrical currents in the mouths of people with amalgam fillings. Raue has noted that these sufferers do not normally consult their dentists because their complaints do not seem to be related to their teeth, while physicians will treat them symptomatically as they are usually unaware of the cause. Even worse, frequently they are seen as hypochondriacs and neurotics (Raue).

Copper in tap water is another form of metal poisoning which most physicians fail to diagnose. Jennifer Sharp has written of her experience with copper poisoning which began when she moved into an old mansion. Not long after the move, she began to note feelings of tiredness and a 'cloud over my head' as well as headaches, a rumbling stomach and irregular heartbeats – symptoms which she and her husband attributed to stress. Later she developed diarrhea and consulted her doctor but, despite medications, her symptoms worsened and she began to experience symptoms of sudden panic.

Hospitalized for evaluation, she had further blood tests, stool cultures and x-rays as well as a fiber optics exam and a stomach biopsy. All that was found was a very irritable lower colon. Since the evaluation failed to find any evidence of a disease which would explain her symptoms, her doctor decided that her problem must be psychological and referred her for marital counseling.

One thousand dollars later, Jennifer was no better, so she decided to give up on counseling as well as on her doctor. Her condition continued to slowly worsen, but one day she got a clue to the cause of her strange malady by observing her puppy. Like Jennifer, her puppy had had diarrhea since she had gotten her. She had not made a connection with her illness as her puppy was unlikely to have contracted her 'mental illness'; worms was the more likely diagnosis. She now noticed, however, that there was a blue-green ring developing around her puppy's water bowl. To be safe, she had the water tested by a local company.

The report was not terribly helpful. The water was acid (pH 5.9) and had some copper in it (1,400 micrograms per liter). Since the acceptable limit of copper is 1,000 micrograms, the results were suspicious, but far from definitive. She then sent a sample of her hair for a mineral analysis which showed her hair copper to be above the suspicious range. She now began to work with an environmental toxicologist who had the state laboratory test the water from the faucet after it had been sitting all night. This time the result was 7,300 micrograms!

Treatment was started after further tests confirmed her

elevated tissue levels of copper. Improvement since then has been slow but steady (Sharp).

FOOD AND CHEMICAL SENSITIVITY

It is frightening to think that environmental substances can produce varied and bizarre symptomatology which second line physicians will frequently dismiss as examples of nondisease. Even more unsettling is the evidence that environmental substances do not have to be toxic to produce devastating physical and mental symptoms. Ordinary foods, even foods considered to be especially nutritious, can be responsible for symptoms in susceptible people. Chemicals in our environment which are non-toxic to most people at the usual levels of exposure can also be responsible.

The field which devotes itself to the diagnosis and treatment of such substance sensitivities is clinical ecology. Its roots are in the field of allergy, although it is unclear how often these sensitivities are allergic in origin. A highly controversial field, part of the controversy is due to differing definitions of what constitutes an allergic reaction.

'Allergy' was introduced in 1906 by von Piquet to describe an 'altered reaction' to tuberculin and soon became the standard term for an altered reaction to a normally innocuous substance to which the individual had been exposed. Further research demonstrated that some of these altered reactions could be traced to specific immunological changes and, as early as 1926, the proposal was made that the term 'allergy' be restricted to reactions which could be shown to reflect changes in immune responses. Most allergists agreed, since the identification of the mechanism of action of immunologic reactions provided a specific etiology and gave the field a more scientific base – which, in turn, elevated their stature in the medical community. Besides which, researchers in immunology discovered an extraordinarily complex system of immunoregulation; mastery of the field of clinical immunology was enough of an undertaking without attempting to be involved with reactions whose mechanisms were unknown.

While the medical schools were quick to redefine the field of allergy along immunologic lines, some practicing allergists opposed the change. Many of their patients had no known immunologic abnormalities. When exposed to certain substances, however, these patients became ill. Furthermore, these physicians had developed procedures for treating such patients which were often effective in relieving their symptoms. Abandoning their patients simply because they lacked identified immunopathology was unthinkable.

The split between the two groups of allergists broadened even further in the ensuing years. While the immunologists made rapid advances in their understanding of immunologic mechanisms, the other, much smaller, group found that many of their patients were suffering from symptoms provoked by exposure, not only to natural products, but also to man-made chemicals which were becoming increasingly common in the environment (Randolph); thus, while the immunologists had narrowed their field, these physicians had broadened their field still further.

Finally, in 1965, this latter group officially defined itself by forming an organization, currently named the American Academy of Environmental Medicine, devoted to 'clinical ecology'. The term 'ecology' alluded to the fact that the organization was concerned with the attempt of the organism to adapt to the substances present in its environment.

Clinical ecologists claim that the symptoms produced by these environmental substances are almost as varied as are the substances themselves. 'Classical' allergic reactions produce one or more of a small list of conditions – rhinitis (runny nose), asthma, conjunctivitis, sinusitis, urticaria (hives) and eczema being some of the most common. The foods and chemicals tested by the clinical ecologists, on the other hand, are claimed by them to produce many additional symptoms; in fact, they claim that environmental senstivities can provoke symptoms referable to *all* the systems of the body – including the brain! This is only a partial list, taken from *Tracking Down Hidden Food Allergy* by William G. Crook, M.D. (Jackson, Tenn., Professional Books, 1978):

Physical Symptoms

Head:

Headaches, faintness, dizziness, feeling of fullness in

the head, excessive drowsiness or sleepiness soon after eating, insomnia

Eyes, Ears, Nose and Throat:

Runny nose, stuffy nose, excessive mucous formation, watery eyes, blurring of vision, ringing of the ears, earache, fullness in the ears, fluid in the middle ear, hearing loss, recurrent ear infections, itching ear, ear drainage, sore throats, chronic cough, gagging, canker sores, itching of the roof of the mouth, recurrent sinusitis.

Heart and Lungs:

Palpitations, increased heart rate, rapid heart rate (tachycardia), asthma, congestion in the chest, hoarseness.

Gastrointestinal:

Nausea, vomiting diarrhea, constipation, bloating after meals, belching, colitis, flatulence (passing gas), feeling of fullness in the stomach long after finishing a meal, abdominal pains or cramps.

Skin:

Hives, rashes, eczema, dermatitis, pallor.

Other Symptoms:

Chronic fatigue, weakness, muscle aches and pains, joint aches and pains, swelling of the hands, feet or ankles, urinary tract symptoms (frequency, urgency), vaginal itching, vaginal discharge, hunger (and its close ally, 'binge or spree' eating).

Psychological Symptoms

Anxiety, 'panic attacks,' depression, 'crying jags,' aggressive behavior, irritability, mental dullness, mental lethargy, confusion, excessive daydreaming, hyperactivity, restlessness, learning disabilities, poor work habits, slurred speech, stuttering, inability to concentrate, indifference.

With so marked a difference in orientation, it is hardly surprising that there are major differences in diagnostic and treatment methods between the two groups. Immunologists limit themselves to diagnostic tests which detect immunologic changes. The backbone of their treatment of allergy is immunotherapy, a technique which dates back to 1911. It is a procedure of limited efficacy, requiring a patient to have a series of sometimes uncomfortable injections weekly, often for years, in the hope of producing some decrease in the severity of the allergic symptoms.

Most fascinating of the techniques employed by the clinical ecologists, and one of the most controversial, is a procedure by which patients are 'neutralized' to foods and chemicals. In this procedure, a series of dilutions of extracts of a suspected substance are either injected into the skin or placed beneath the tongue. If symptoms develop or, in the case of the injections, if the wheal which forms shows at least 2 millimeters growth in ten minutes, the test is considered to indicate that the patient is sensitive to that substance. Other dilutions of the extract are then administered in an attempt to find a dilution which will 'neutralize' or remove the symptoms. When neutralization is successful, the patient is provided with a supply of that dilution and instructed to use it to prevent reactions to the substance.

There is no doubt that there are many satisfied patients who are delighted to attest to the efficacy of clinical ecologic procedures. Some of them have even formed their own organization for the purpose of sharing information concerning food and chemical sensitivities and of fostering the acceptance of such concepts (Human Ecology Action League). The majority of physicians, on the other hand, citing the absence of proven mechanisms by which these often bizarre symptoms are mediated, contend that these symptoms are simply expressions of the patients' unconscious minds and thus that any benefits they derive from treatments are merely due to placebo effects (Nelson).

Is there any scientific evidence to back up the assertions of clinical ecology? The answer is yes – although so far the evidence is only limited and fragmentary. There are, for example, double-blind studies in the literature which have demonstrated improvement in hyperactive children on an elimination diet with worsening upon challenge with certain of the eliminated foods (Egger *et al.* 1985), while other double-blind studies have demonstrated that treatment with food extracts can be associated with significant behavioral improvements in hyperactive children (Rapp, O'Shea and Porter).

In addition to demonstrating a relationship between food sensitivities and hyperactivity, double-blind studies have demonstrated an important relationship between food sensitivities and symptoms of migraine headaches (Egger *et al.*, 1983, Monro *et al.*), irritable bowel syndrome (Jones *et al.*) and rheumatoid arthritis (Mandell and Conte, Marshall *et al.*). In addition, there are published case reports of people who became ill with the multiple symptoms described by clinical ecologists following heavy exposures to environmental chemicals whose immune systems showed abnormalities. When they were re-exposed to those chemicals under double-blind conditions, not only were their symptoms reactivated, but their immune systems also reacted (Rea *et al.* 1978).

One double-blind study has demonstrated that foods and chemicals can produce both cognitive and emotional symptoms when administered as extracts under the tongue (King), while others have demonstrated the efficacy of intradermal neutralization (Boris *et al.*, Miller, Rea *et al.*, 1984).

The *Lancet* has published a series of case reports which also support the concept of a multi-system involvement in food sensitivities. Two of these cases are particularly noteworthy. The first was of a man with severe episodic pain in his right iliac fossa. A tube was inserted through his nose into his stomach so he could not identify what was being given to him. Tea or water was given via the tube in an irregular sequence on five different occasions. Each time tea was given he immediately developed a rapid heart beat and developed his abdominal pain the next day – but no reaction occurred when water was given.

The other case was of a woman with severe nausea and vomiting. Tea, but not water, when delivered through the tube, produced vomiting within thirty minutes. For both of these patients, the statistical probability of their reactions occurring by chance is only 1 to 1024 (Finn and Cohen).

There is even reason to believe that we may be close to establishing a scientific explanation for the development of cognitive and emotional symptoms from the ingestion of food. It is beginning to appear that the brain requires a certain level of endorphins to function normally (Verebey *et al.*). Schizophrenics, for example, have been found to have endorphin levels ten times those of normals (Domschke *et al.*). Strange as it seems, fractions of milk (casein) and wheat (gluten) have recently been found to have morphine-like activity, and could conceivably be absorbed from the gut in certain circumstances and cross through the blood-brain barrier into the brain where they would have direct effects upon brain function (Zioudrou *et al.*). This may explain the finding that some acute schizophrenics improve more rapidly when they are placed on a milk-free and cereal-free diet (Dohan and Grasberger).

Obviously, not all of us develop mental symptoms from drinking milk or eating wheat. Reasons why only some people are so affected are just becoming clear. Secretory immunoglobulin A, for example, appears to act as a barrier for food antigens passing from the gut into the circulation (Cunningham-Rubdles *et al.*). People who have low levels of secretory IgA, therefore, may introduce a higher than normal level of undigested or partly digested food into their bloodstreams, causing both direct effects from their morphine-like activities and indirect effects from their challenge to the immune system. Indeed, some people with food sensitivities have been found to have depressed levels of this immunoglobulin (McGovern *et al.*). Furthermore, clinical ecologists have long noted that food sensitivities often start after a period of stress, and recently stress has been shown to lower secretory IgA levels (Jemmott *et al.*).

CANDIDA ALBICANS OVERGROWTH

Another cause for food sensitivities which was undiscovered until the past few years is overgrowth of candida albicans, a yeast which normally inhabits the bowel and produces no symptoms. It is well known that people in terminal stages of illnesses may develop fulminating yeast infections as their immune defenses crumble, but it had been thought that, other than producing symptoms directly related to obvious yeast infections, candida lives quite happily within us without even causing illness.

Evidence is mounting, however, that candida is responsible for a multitude of systemic symptoms even though there is no evidence of the yeast reaching the blood stream. These are thought to include:

gastrointestinal symptoms:
- bloating
- flatus (gas)
- diarrhea

pruritis (itchiness)
anxiety or irritability
depression
tiredness
premenstrual syndrome

Afflicted patients often have a history of recurrent athlete's foot or fungal infections of the nails. Symptoms commonly began following courses of antibiotics or steroids, or in women, following pregnancy, the use of female hormones, or the development of vaginal yeast infections.

As is the case with many hidden causes of multisystem illnesses, the discovery that candida albicans was responsible for such varied symptoms was an empirical one. C. Orion Truss, an internist and allergist, discovered the connection when he found that many of his patients with suspicious histories and no other medical explanation for their symptoms responded dramatically to anti-fungal drugs (Truss 1982 and 1984, Crook). Until recently, the diagnosis could only be made on the basis of a positive response to treatment, but now laboratory testing for anti-candida antibodies is becoming available to assist clinicians by providing an objective basis for evaluating patients. Since nearly everyone has some candida in his or her body, and therefore some degree of antibody response, this test compares the level of anti-candida antibodies to that of the normal population.

The scientific verification of such a syndrome is still only preliminary, although interest in candida has grown to the point that a Yeast-Human Interaction Conference is held annually in the United States to provide an opportunity for experts in relevant clinical and research areas to discuss their latest findings (For information, write to: Critical Illness Research Foundation, 2614 Highland Avenue, Birmingham, Alabama 35205).

NASOPHARYNGEAL INFLAMMATION

The average layman is well aware of how to diagnose the common cold, but even second line physicians are generally unaware that a mild degree of chronic inflammation in a particular region of the throat can be responsible for a number of well-known illnesses. This region, called the nasopharynx, is located behind the nose and above the region of the throat which is visible behind the mouth (the oropharynx). Its importance is due to the fact that the sphenopalatine ganglion lies in close proximity. A part of the sympathetic nervous system, the sphenopalatine ganglion contains the largest collection of neurons in the head outside of the brain and has extensive connections with major nerves, another major sympathetic ganglion and the aggregation of nerve fibers surrounding the internal carotid artery on its way to the brain.

During a cold, most people will notice a dry feeling in the back of the roof of the mouth (the soft palate). This sensation is associated with acute nasopharyngitis. Chronic nasopharyngitis, by contrast, has no obvious signs or symptoms which would call attention to it. Moreover, the nasopharynx is impossible to view without special equipment, so that it is usually ignored – even by otolaryngologists.

Sinsak Horiguti, Professor Emeritus of the Tokyo Medical and Dental University, has published numerous articles in the professional literature documenting the relationship between inflammation of the nasopharynx and disorders of the autonomic nervous system. These disorders include:

vertigo
hypertension
gastric ulcers
asthma
hypotension
migraine headaches
constipation
diarrhea
palpitations

Diagnosis and treatment is remarkably simple. Severe pain is noted when the physician brushes the nasopharynx with a cotton-tipped applicator. Local treatment by abrasion or the application of medications results in prompt healing with disappearance of the associated disorder (Horiguti).

Asa Ruskin, Associate Clinical Professor of Rehabilitation Medicine at Albert Einstein College of Medicine has reviewed the literature on treating autonomic nervous disorders by anesthetizing the sphenopalatine ganglion which is located adjacent to the nasopharynx. As with Horiguti's work, excellent results have been reported in the same disorders, which suggests that nasopharyngeal irritation may cause distant symptoms due to its effect upon the ganglion. Results have also been excellent when the technique has been applied to the treatment of a variety of chronic pain syndromes (Ruskin).

Patients can indeed present with a syndrome which mimics a known disease – or even with a bizarre collection of symptoms accompanied by few or no clinical signs of disease. Second Line Medicine, with its strict divisions, textbook orientation and mind-body dichotomization, has relegated these people to psychiatric care. Such a referral is often inappropriate, for an actual disease may be present, even though second line physicians are poorly equipped to discover it.

Following appropriate evaluations by medical specialists, these patients can be best treated by third line physicians. The search for occult disease can then continue. The possibility of a psychological cause for the symptoms can be assessed without the psychological bias inherent in Second Line medicine towards patients without proven disease.

Clifton Meader, in elucidating the concept of nondisease, has wondered 'how many . . . unrecognized nondiseases are still being treated as diseases today.' (Meader).

My question is the opposite: how many unrecognized *diseases* are still being treated as nondiseases?

CHAPTER 10
The quest for health: journeys through the system

> The physician
> is nature's assistant.
>
> GALEN
> 2nd century AD

The experience of illness is universal – yet the journey each of us embarks upon when we become ill is a lonely one, for each of us has a unique constitution and history which separates us from our brethren. Individuality is lost, however, when our stories become compressed with those of others to form group statistics. These statistics tell us much about common characteristics, but nothing about individual ones which vary from the average. Thus, if we wish to select an appropriate treatment for an individual, group statistics may be misleading.

On the other hand, single case experimental designs are also inadequate, as they only provide data about an isolated characteristic of an individual. Since other individuals who share that characteristic still differ in many other ways, there is no way of knowing if they will show the same results as the experimental subject. Even at best, scientific data can only *suggest* that an individual may respond to a specific treatment; the practice of medicine offers no guarantees.

Astute clinicians first become familiar with their patients. Next they review the scientific literature to gather leads. Lastly, before suggesting treatments, they review their personal experience with similar patients as well as the personal experiences of other clinicians. These personal experiences, formally called *anecdotal case reports*, fill in some of the gaps left by science.

I offer the following anecdotal case reports in order to give the flavor of Third Line Medicine. As with any medical treatment, cases can be selected to show either good or poor results. These are selected more because they illustrate the art and challenge of Third Line Medicine than because of their outcome. Names and other specifics have been changed to preserve the patients' anonymity.

THE CASE OF THE SPINNING ROOM

Jan, a businesswoman in her early thirties, was fully disabled when she first consulted me. In addition to a constant feeling of malaise, about once a week her head would start to feel 'full'. Shortly afterwards, she would hear a high-pitched ringing which would be followed, one or two days later, by an episode of vertigo. The vertigo, in turn, would be followed by nausea, and then by vomiting. After throwing up, Jan would fall asleep and later awaken wet with perspiration and relieved of all of her symptoms except the feeling of malaise.

She initially consulted an otologist. Her tests were normal and he placed her on a vasodilator (medication to enlarge her blood vessels) which did little to help her symptoms. She continued to see him when her symptoms flared up; at one point he discovered diminished hearing in one ear and diagnosed her as suffering from Meniere's Syndrome. Since he had no more to offer her, he referred her to a sub-specialist who performed a battery of tests which revealed an abnormality in the left inner ear as well as reactive hypoglycemia.

She decided to consult a specialist in hypoglycemia (despite the objection of her internist). Even though she was slender, he put her on a diet whose only effect was to cause her to lose weight until she weighed just ninety-three pounds. Meanwhile, her otologist started her on further medications and vitamins which was followed by a temporary remission. Her condition gradually worsened, however, until her otologist suggested surgery.

She then sought a second opinion. While the consultant agreed that surgery might be necessary, he noted that her condition was common in young executives who are under a great deal of tension. She returned to her otologist who advised allergy testing prior to proceeding with surgery. As testing revealed multiple allergies, he recommended that she return to her internist for a trial of immunotherapy, a treatment which her internist believed to be valueless to her. Instead, he referred her to me for a consultation.

Jan's background intrigued me. As a child, she had been repeatedly rejected by parental figures. Her father left her mother shortly after her birth and, until recently, she had never met him. She was raised by her mother's parents who favored her brother and gave her attention only when she was ill. When she was thirteen, her mother remarried and moved out of the area, taking her brother with her. Later Jan was placed with neighbors so that her grandparents could move to Florida. Feeling abandoned, she obtained a one-way ticket to Florida by convincing her uncle that her grandparents had invited her to come for a visit. Her plan worked. Since her grandparents could not afford to send her back, they permitted her to remain with them in Florida.

At age fifteen, Jan became ill with cystitis. Her grandparents had had enough, so they sent her to live with her mother and step-father. Her step-father was less than enthusiastic over taking responsibility for her; he punished her severely for the slightest infractions of his rules.

Jan married before she was eighteen. By age nineteen, she had divorced her husband and remarried. Eight years later, Jan had become fed up with her husband's 'parasitic dependency' and, despite his protests, filed for divorce. This period, according to her, was the most upsetting time of her life. It was also the time that the ringing began in her ears.

Jan was intelligent, attractive and charming but her smile seemed incongruous with the distressing history which she reported. Psychological testing suggested that she had a strong need to rationalize her anger and predicted that she could become increasingly incapacitated by physical symptoms which were prompted by hidden emotional responses.

I suggested a treatment program which consisted of both biofeedback-assisted relaxation training sessions and psychodynamic psychotherapy. Jan agreed and, over the next few months, she received a total of twenty sessions of biofeedback training along with an equal number of psychotherapy sessions. In the biofeedback sessions, I taught her to relax her body with the aid of two biofeedback instruments while, in the psychotherapy sessions, we explored her reactions to past and current stresses.

Following the first biofeedback session, she no longer experienced nausea during her attacks. Her tinnitus, which had been constant for eight days, suddenly vanished while she was driving home from her second biofeedback session. It reappeared a few more times, but each episode was milder than the previous one. Similarly, her vertigo rapidly subsided. By the seventeenth session, Jan was totally asymptomatic for the first time in 4½ years.

Her ratings of depression did not coincide with her ratings of her physical symptoms. Since Jan had attributed her depression to her disability, she was perplexed when she suddenly began to feel more depressed, restless and irritable once her physical symptoms began to subside. Insomnia developed and she began to lose her temper and scream at her family – even though she believed that screaming was improper. She also began to assert herself more strongly to her family and friends despite her fear that now she would be rejected by them because of her 'bitchiness'. In fact, Jan was now faced with discovering whether her husband and children really cared for her, or whether they just liked her because she had been acting so pleasant and charming. After her childhood experiences, she did not really want to find out.

Fortunately, her husband and children came through for her. By this time, she was married to her third husband and was mother to five children. They were concerned about the striking changes in her behavior, but they were caring and supportive. As a result, Jan felt reassured and her depression rapidly subsided. Jan had learned at an early age that her expression of unpleasant feelings caused her to be rejected. Illness had become the only acceptable way of gaining the attention and support she needed from others. Now, for the first time, Jan learned that she could trust her family with her feelings – and discovered that they loved her.

I wish her story ended here; however, more stresses were to come. Jan remained free of all symptoms for six months. Then her mother came to town to visit her for a week. While her mother was visiting, Jan developed an acute attack of bronchial asthma. The attack soon ended and she went on vacation with her husband to a resort to recuperate only to have a second attack at the resort. When the second attack ended, the ringing in her ears returned. She practiced the relaxation procedures she had learned and the ringing ceased after four days – but was immediately followed by the onset of incapacitating low back pain which lasted several days.

The following week Jan enrolled in a behavioral program to stop smoking without first consulting me. The program trained her to experience nausea whenever she thought of smoking. She began to hear ringing again on the last day of the five-day program. One month later, shortly after attempting to mediate between two people who were threatening to sue one another, she began to feel nauseated and the entire Meniere's Syndrome returned, but with one difference. This time nausea was the most predominant symptom.

Jan returned to me for a few additional biofeedback sessions to try to regain the control she had achieved. She was too nauseated, however, to relax well. Rather than return to psychotherapy, which I believe would have helped her, she soon gave up hope and dropped out.

Comments

Jan's case illustrates the importance of understanding and dealing with the psychological contribution to physical symptoms as well as the benefits of combining treatment modalities. When psychological issues are major contributors to physical symptoms, especially when those symptoms are associated with hyperactivation of the autonomic nervous system, relaxation training is often faster than dynamic psychotherapy in achieving symptom reduction. The procedure may, however, need to be offered in conjunction with psychotherapy for patients who will need assistance in coping with the thoughts and feelings which may arise when their bodily symptoms subside.

We can only speculate as to the reasons why Jan's case history, after all that she had accomplished, ended on a note of failure. I suspect that Jan had regressed to her former habit of hiding her feelings during her mother's visit with the result that her old defense of converting those feelings into physical symptoms returned. With all of her assets, I am hopeful that she continued to work through her problems after she left my care. If so, I am optimistic that she could reach the point where her life would no longer be burdened by unnecessary physical ailments.

THE CASE OF THE MYSTERIOUS PAIN ATTACKS

Linda's illness began without warning one morning when, upon awakening, she suddenly experienced a strange, cool sensation over part of her face which was mildly painful. The sensation soon left her but returned another day and gradually increased in its frequency, severity and area of distribution. She eventually sought the aid of her internist. He referred her to a neurologist who found nothing on his initial exam to explain her symptoms. He then ordered a full battery of studies including skull x-rays, an EEG (brain wave tracing) and a brain scan, all of which failed to reveal any abnormalities. Since she also had a history of headaches which seemed to be migrainous, he decided to start her on cyproheptadine, a histamine and serotonin antagonist. The drug helped her headaches but had no effect on her facial pain.

In taking Linda's history, the neurologist found that she had been going through a period of considerable stress. Her daughter not only had headaches like hers, but also had had a recent episode during which she lost consciousness and had a seizure. After her daughter's seizure, Linda's facial pains were worse, and she also lost her appetite. The neurologist concluded that her facial pains were 'a conversion problem;' i.e. that she was unconsciously expressing her feelings through imagined sensory changes in her face.

Linda was not satisfied with his diagnosis, so she sought the services of another physician. He thought that her sensation of coolness might be due to spasm of the blood vessels and prescribed niacin. Unfortunately, the niacin was ineffective. Yet another physician was consulted, and again he failed to suggest anything which brought her relief. After four years of searching, she began a program of acupuncture. At first she felt considerable improvement but, after fifty acupuncture sessions, she found she was back to where she had started.

After six years, Linda went to see another neurologist who, once again, could find no evidence of an organic cause for her facial pain. He felt that he had nothing to offer her, since he was convinced that she did not have organic disease, and suggested that she see me for a consultation.

I found Linda to be a pleasant and intelligent woman of menopausal age who appeared neither anxious nor depressed but was clearly frustrated over the failure of her doctors to find an effective treatment for what had become an increasingly severe pain syndrome. By now, her pain was becoming almost unbearable. On a scale of one to ten, where one represents a slight discomfort and ten represents unbearable pain, she stated that her pain was reaching nine. It was a constant pain over most of her face as well as her ears and part of her neck. The episodes would occur anytime without warning, from daily to as rarely as a few times a month. They were unrelated to heat, cold, emotional or physical distress or the season of the year. She continued to have occasional migraine headaches, but these were much less frequent since she was placed on propanolol.

I probed her for a possible psychological cause to explain her symptom. She was most cooperative, but we could find no clues from her history other than the fact that her husband had had a heart attack three years earlier which had made her worry about his health. She noted that she often had an attack of facial pain not long after he left for work – a fact which she thought might indicate that her worry over his health bore some relationship to the syndrome, even though the onset of the pain seemed to be unrelated to what she was thinking at the moment.

Despite this information, I was not convinced that her pain was psychogenic. Linda seemed to be too healthy psychologically to have developed such a severe pain syndrome because of inability to cope with her husband's heart condition. I gave her a psychological test (MMPI) which confirmed my impression. Her psychological profile was essentially normal and her ego strength, or general coping abilities, was much above average.

I then questioned whether her pain could be due to some type of hyperactivation syndrome wherein normal structures might become overactivated from some unidentified stimulus to produce pain. To assess this possibility, I attached her to physiologic monitoring instruments and found her to display no evidence of hyperactivation. Since the physiologic readings were taken when she had no pain, I asked her to call me during an episode and arrange to see me immediately so that I could see if she showed a hyperactivation pattern at that time. She did so, and once again she showed no evidence of excessive physiologic activity which could explain her severe level of pain.

I then performed a brief trial of electrical acupuncture. These succeeded in decreasing the area of pain, but had no effect on its frequency or intensity. I was convinced that I was missing something, but what? Earlier I had reviewed her allergic history which was negative. Now, however, as we searched for additional historical clues, Linda revealed that two years ago her skin had broken out in an itchy rash which cleared up as soon as she stopped her multivitamin.

Perhaps Linda was food sensitive! She noted that her syndrome worsened soon after her husband's heart attack. While earlier she thought that perhaps it had worsened because of the stress, she now recalled that, after his heart attack, they stopped eating eggs each morning to cut down on cholesterol. Instead they began to eat a daily bowl of raisin bran. Could something in the cereal be causing the pain?

We decided to try a five-day fast during which she drank only spring water. By 10 am on the first morning of the fast she began to note facial pain which gradually worsened until it became severe and she became nauseated. Later in the day she developed what she described as the worst migraine in her life which persisted until the fourth day. On the second day she noted muscular pains in her thighs and calves which gradually faded away. On the fourth day she had a second attack of facial pain which was much milder but persisted all day. By the fifth day she was feeling fine except for hunger. Linda had been through the classical withdrawal syndrome described for masked food sensitivities!

We began to slowly return foods to her diet. She had no

symptoms until a few hours after adding wheat when she had a typical episode of facial pain. We removed wheat from her diet and gradually added back all other foods without incurring any further episodes of pain.

Since then, Linda has usually been free of all facial pain. Occasionally, between thirty minutes and four hours after ingesting a food, she develops her pain syndrome. When this occurs, she attempts to discover the exact ingredients of that food. Invariably, she finds that one of those ingredients was wheat.

Comments

Linda's case illustrates the folly of assuming that symptoms which cannot be shown to be accompanied by physical changes are necessarily psychological in origin when, in fact, they may have a physical cause which routine procedures are unable to demonstrate. Even worse, the statement that a symptom is psychogenic carries such negative connotations in our society that it often justifies a dismissal of treatment efforts as well as of third party insurance coverage to pay for those efforts.

THE CASE OF THE WOMAN WHO WOULD NO LONGER STAND FOR IT

Glenda, a married woman in her early sixties, was referred due to a two-year history of progressive fatiguability in her legs associated with throbbing and numbness which started after a bout of influenza. A comprehensive neurological evaluation at a university medical center failed to find evidence of a physical lesion which could explain her symptoms.

She had been married almost forty years and described her marriage as 'fair'. While her husband was a kind and well-meaning person, she noted that he had always been unable to take any leadership in the marriage; thus she had reluctantly been forced to take a leadership role. To make matters worse, several years ago he had suffered a stroke which left him less sharp mentally. She complained that she was always having to lead him in recent years and was unable to have meaningful conversations with him. She had become depressed about her marriage at times but saw no way out as she would feel too guilty if she left him. In fact, just prior to the onset of her symptoms, she had been agitated over her husband's deficits in judgment and foresight.

Since her symptoms began, she was feeling tense, irritable and moderately depressed – symptoms which she attributed to her reaction to her illness. Sexual activity with her husband was minimal because 'I'm so numb that I don't feel a reaction.' She was no longer feeling angry at him, however, as her concerns had shifted from the marriage to her physical symptoms and disability, a disability which forced him to assume more responsibility in the marriage.

Psychological testing suggested that her psychological problems fell into the neurotic range. Depression was the dominant feature along with feelings of inadequacy, sexual conflict, rigidity, chronic anxiety, fatigue and tension. She appeared to be overconcerned about her bodily functions and physical health and could be experiencing 'fatigue, weakness and generalized aches and pains without clear organic etiology.'

Glenda agreed to a series of ten sessions of biofeedback-assisted relaxation training. Her muscle tension was not unduly high and most of her readings fell within the normal range. Her finger temperature was moderately cool (which was evidence that at least part of her nervous system was not relaxed) and she was unable to learn to warm her fingers. Her level of skin conductance (another indicator of the level of activation of the autonomic nervous system) was extremely low and unresponsive to both physical and emotional stimuli, so low that, on two occasions, I was unable even to get a reading. This pattern has been shown to correlate to depression. Glenda was cooperative and attempted to utilize the exercises I taught her yet, strangely enough, she was unable to learn to discriminate even major differences in the level of tension in her body.

After ten training sessions, she reported that her symptoms were no better. 'I'm reaching the conclusion', she lamented, 'that my mind is my worst enemy. I feel very responsible for my family.' We reviewed her family situation and she was able to accept the possibility that her mind had created her disability as the only solution which would be acceptable to her, given her moral values and her ambivalent feelings towards her husband. Only by becoming disabled could her dependency needs be met; she had no other option. She did not wish psychotherapy as she believed that she was already aware of the psychodynamic issues and did not see how psychotherapy would help her to find a healthier solution.

Six months after that meeting, I called Glenda to ask how she was doing. She reported that, since her last session with me, she had undergone trials of bioenergetics and hypnosis. Her symptoms, however, had continued to progress.

Comments

Glenda's case illustrates the powerful effect which psychological conflicts can have upon the body. Sometimes the enhanced awareness people experience when they learn the relaxation response leads them to discover a better solution to their conflicts by themselves; other times the enhanced awareness along with the aid of an experienced psychotherapist leads them to a better solution. For Glenda, however, there was no better solution. She could not live with the guilt she would feel if she left her husband, yet she could not live with her husband unless she somehow found a means by which she could get him to gratify her unfulfilled dependency wishes. Her disability was her unconscious solution. Unfortunately, I could not offer her a better one which she would find acceptable.

THE CASE OF THE MAN WHO KEPT PASSING OUT

Greg's injury occurred more than three years before I first saw him. He reported that he had slipped at work and had fallen flat on his back. Because of back pain, he was admitted to the hopsital where he began to note aching pains in the back of his neck which radiated forward 'like they were pushing my eye out'. While the backache subsided, the headaches did not and, despite visits to numerous doctors, their pattern failed to change over time.

He told me that his headaches were occurring a couple of times a week and lasting a few hours. They would awaken him from sleep or occur randomly during the day without warning and would start with a 'kink' in the neck. During the headache the area around his eyes would swell. At times he could end an attack by going to sleep. Otherwise only a combination of a major tranquilizer and an antidepressant seemed to give any relief – but these medications drugged him so badly that he could 'barely feel anything' when he took them.

His 'blackouts' began around the same time as the headaches even though they had no regular relationship with them. Like the headaches, they seemed to occur randomly. According to a witness, he would suddenly fall forward without warning. Sometimes he would injure himself when he fell and, in fact, had recently broken his front teeth from one of his falls.

The diagnosis of his headaches had varied from doctor to doctor. Two thought he had migraine headaches which were unrelated to his injury. One thought he had sprained neck muscles, while another concluded that he probably had a pinched nerve. Nobody could explain his blackouts on the basis of physical or laboratory findings. As his injury was covered under the Worker's Compensation laws, and he first reported the blackouts to physicians months after the injury, his physicians were suspicious that his complaints, if they existed at all, occurred because of psychological, rather than physical, factors. A psychiatrist concluded that Greg had a Passive-Aggressive Personality with repressed hostility which was expressed through the body as tension headaches. A neurologist stated that he had a Post-Traumatic Psychoneurosis while a second psychiatrist found no evidence of psychiatric illness. A second neurologist called his fainting spells 'neurotic'. A third psychiatrist agreed with the first that he had a Passive-Aggressive Personality and considered his spells to be unexplainable. A third neurologist called the spells 'psychogenic' and a fourth psychiatrist stated that Greg was simply lying about his symptoms as he was not motivated to return to work.

I was the fifth psychiatrist. When Greg came into my office he sank so deeply into the chair that I immediately doubted that his headaches were the usual muscle contraction headaches which tense people are prone to develop. In fact, just looking at him slumping in the chair, I could see how his attitude could be easily interpreted as angry and he could be viewed as being lazy. I decided to arrange for neuropsychologic testing in order to rule out a subtle degree of brain damage as well as psychologic testing in order to see if it substantiated the psychiatric diagnoses he had been given.

Both tests failed to find any evidence of an abnormality. I hooked him up to my biofeedback equipment, but could find no evidence of hyperactivation as a cause of his headaches. In fact, I found his heart rate to be unusually low, in the range of forty-four to fifty-three beats per minute. Assuming that Greg really did suffer from his stated complaints, how, then could I explain them? A novel thought came to mind. Since Greg was so relaxed, perhaps his fainting spells were due to an abnormally *low* level of activation of the autonomic nervous system. His headaches, then, could be his attempt to keep alert by tensing his muscles!

If my hypothesis were true, we could treat Greg's symptoms by teaching him to increase his activation in more effective ways while teaching him to avoid tensing his neck and scalp muscles. Greg agreed to work with me and my staff on this goal, so we began a program of biofeedback-assisted arousal training. Our baseline was the two weeks prior to starting training during which he reported two fainting spells each week. We taught him to increase both his heart rate and his level of skin conductance while simultaneously maintaining a low level of muscle tension. During the week following his first session, he had only one fainting spell. Then he had no spells for the next six weeks!

One day, however, after digging ditches, he suddenly fainted on a staircase, fell down the stairs and was hospitalized briefly with a concussion. Afterwards we worked with Greg for three more months during which time he reported no fainting spells. He was expressing interest in returning to work by the time that we terminated. Except for an occasional headache, he was feeling fine.

Comments

When physical findings are absent, it is all too easy for

physicians to conclude that symptoms are either willfully falsified or caused by psychological problems. I prefer to attempt to see symptoms from the patient's perspective – and reach such conclusions only after I have found adequate data to substantiate them.

THE CASE OF THE FOUR FAILED FUSIONS

Alice was referred from a university low back pain clinic due to a ten-year history of low back pain unrelieved by treatment. She was a young, married secretary who had become fully disabled due to an auto accident. Initially medications and physical therapy were tried, but she failed to respond, so she received a laminectomy and a fusion. After surgery, her pain was worse than ever. When, after three years of conservative treatment, her pain was no better, a second fusion was performed, but the results were again unsuccessful. She next received a series of acupuncture treatments without benefit and, the following year, a third fusion was performed. Once again, she failed to improve.

Transcutaneous nerve stimulation, massage and other non-surgical procedures were then tried, but her pain persisted at the same level. She then received her *fourth* fusion. This time she was placed in a body cast for ten months after surgery. Afterwards she was somewhat better, but remained in considerable distress. Nerve blocks were tried, but she only achieved pain relief while her legs were paralyzed from the anesthetic.

She had been evaluated by a psychiatrist, but he found no evidence of significant psychological problems. She then saw a psychologist who taught her some hypnotic relaxation techniques which relieved the pain, but only temporarily.

When I saw Alice for evaluation, she reported that her pain had become increasingly severe since giving birth to two children only about a year apart. She claimed that she was too busy to relax, since the babies, both still in diapers, were very demanding and neither slept through the night. Although the pain was not clearly related to the amount of stress she was under at any particular moment, she noted that she was moderately tense and occasionally depressed. Psychological testing revealed significant depression and a tendency to focus on physical symptoms rather than to admit to or deal directly with emotional problems.

She and I decided on a series of biofeedback-assisted relaxation training sessions. We found that her level of muscle tension was so elevated that we could expect her to feel pain just from muscular contraction. She rapidly learned to decrease these values and was often able to reduce them into the relaxed range by the end of the session. She also became skilful at voluntarily increasing her finger temperature with regularity. In addition, during the sessions, she was open about her stresses at home and it became clear that there were significant marital problems.

After completing ten training sessions, Alice reported that she was so much better that she had been able to discontinue her pain medications. At times she was now free of pain although, at other times, the pain could be as severe as it had ever been. In addition, she was much better able to cope with and tolerate the pain.

Repeated psychological testing also showed improvement, although she still appeared to be moderately depressed. Most striking was the reduction of her score for hypochondriasis (fear of disease causing symptoms to be perceived as worse than they need to be) which fell from a highly elevated score all the way to the normal range. We decided that she could benefit from additional sessions.

Alice terminated from the program after completing nineteen training sessions. By then her pain was only mild. The focus of her treatment had gradually shifted from her physical pain to the emotional pain she was experiencing in her marriage. She became aware of her need to work actively on this problem and began marital counseling.

Six months later, we called her to inquire about her progress. She reported that she was continuing to utilize the exercises we had taught her. Her back pain was now even less than it was when she terminated with us.

Two and a half years later, Alice returned. She was still in marital counseling, but had been feeling more stressed for the past year due to a number of family pressures. Her back pain had continued to be minimal but, along with feeling increasingly depressed, she had developed abdominal pain, periodic vomiting, and alternating constipation and diarrhea. A gastroenterologist had evaluated her, concluded that she had a spastic colon, and had prescribed a number of medications for her to try. Strangely enough, the medications only worsened her symptoms. This frustrated her doctor and caused her to feel that he blamed her for not getting better.

This time I did not believe that Alice needed further relaxation training sessions. She was continuing to practice her exercises and her back pain remained minimal, so it was unlikely that her new symptoms were due to an inability to relax. Instead, the symptoms sounded suspicious for the presence of food sensitivities. I asked her whether she had any history of allergies. Sure enough, she reported having frequent sinus infections and bronchitis due to numerous inhalants including tobacco smoke and house dust. I decided to recommend sublingual provocative testing in order to discover if she was, in fact, sensitive to certain foods.

At the testing session, Alice reported experiencing strong stomach cramps as well as nasal stuffiness, headache and sleepiness when we gave her drops of milk extract in a glycerin solution under the tongue. She also reported that she had been developing spontaneous bruises for the past two weeks. I started her on nutritional supplements and, based on the results of provocative testing, had her remove certain foods from her diet.

Two weeks later she reported that she was symptom-free for short intervals for the first time in months. Her abdominal pains were much milder, although she also noted increased gas and diarrhea. She was no longer developing spontaneous bruises. I suggested digestive enzymes for her to take with meals and encouraged her to switch to organic foods as much as possible. When I last heard from her, all her gastrointestinal symptoms had greatly improved. She would occasionally break out in hives, and found that the cause was usually a food.

Comments

Alice's case illustrates the complex nature of bodily symptoms.

Pains are never purely physical and rarely purely psychological; most are influenced by a number of etiological factors of which the psychological state of the individual is only one. If, when physicians identify one factor, they don't stop their attempts to identify other factors, they will have the highest probability of success in benefiting their patients.

THE CASE OF THE MAN LOST IN COMA

Life was going well for Jim, a married engineer in his mid-thirties, when tragedy struck. Deep within his brain, the great cerebral vein of Galen ruptured and Jim collapsed. Twice surgeons opened up his skull and attempted to repair the damage. Shunts were installed to relieve the brain of the pressure it was under from the leak.

Yet, six months later, Jim remained in a deep coma. The rigid posturing of his body indicated that his cerebrum, the cognitive portion of his brain, was not functioning. Because of the danger that he could acquire a fatal infection in his debilitated state, visitors had to put on sterile gowns and face masks before entering his room. He appeared to be more dead than alive. As he was unresponsive to all but physically painful stimuli, the nursing staff made no efforts to relate to him, and acted almost as if the man in the bed were already a corpse.

Jim's family, however, was not ready to give up hope for his recovery. Instead, they called me and asked if there was anything I might be able to do to help him. By coincidence, I had recently heard a talk given by a man who claimed that he had been successful in making contact with coma victims and had even succeeded in guiding some of them out of their comas. While, like most people, I needed more than simply his case reports to be convinced, I was intrigued by his method.

Coma victims tend to be treated as if they are unaware of what is happening around them – even though, unless they have no brainwave activity, we really don't know how much actually registers in their brains. At the time, it had occurred to me that biofeedback instruments might improve the chances of achieving communication although, to the best of my knowledge, they had never been used before for that purpose. The instruments could indicate whether comatose patients were aware that people were talking to them since, if they were aware, their physiological activities might change in response to other people's communications with them. Even more intriguing was the possibility that, if they were in fact conscious but paralyzed, biofeedback instruments could provide a means for them to 'talk'.

Thus, when Jim's family called me, I suggested that, since there was so much to gain and nothing to lose, that I use biofeedback instruments to attempt to achieve communication with Jim. I also suggested that I invite the speaker I had heard to join us and lead the session. They agreed.

We met at Jim's bedside in the hospital where he had been confined for months, surrounded by his immediate family and his nurses. Since the feedback electromyograph (EMG) would convey the slightest changes in the degree of muscle contraction of Jim's voluntary muscles, I attached that machine's electrodes to his forehead. Since changes in the electrical conductance of the skin would indicate the slightest changes in the level of activation of Jim's sympathetic nervous system, I attached galvanic skin response (GSR) electrodes to his fingers.

My associate did most of the speaking while I monitored the biofeedback equipment. He explained to Jim who we were and asked for his cooperation. He then instructed him to focus his attention on one area of his body at a time and to shift his attention from area to area at his signal. During this exercise, I saw no changes on the EMG so I turned it off. Much to my delight, however, the pitch of the feedback GSR started to rise each time my associate asked Jim to shift his focus of attention. We now knew that Jim was hearing us and responding!

Our excitement mounted as my associate asked Jim to focus his attention on his throat. Suddenly, Jim let out a long moan, a moan which continued for several seconds. Jim was communicating!

After the session, we met with Jim's family and I suggested that they arrange for Jim to have another session with my associate. As I did not hear anything further from them, I called Jim's uncle three months later. He reported that my associate had had one more meeting with Jim. By one month after our initial session, Jim was no longer in coma and was discharged to go home with around the clock nursing care. He had gained fifteen pounds and was on the road to further recovery.

Almost exactly two years after our session, I received a telephone call from Jim's mother as she knew I would be interested in hearing of Jim's progress. A year earlier, Jim's parents had moved with him to a rural community so they could concentrate on nursing him back to health. She reported that he was now able to talk in phrases and could feed himself. He required a wheelchair but was able to flex his legs and was continuing to make steady progress. She then called Jim to the phone who told me personally how pleased he was with his progress. Hearing his voice was one of the most rewarding moments I have ever had in the practice of medicine.

Comments

Though we cannot know with certainty whether Jim's recovery was related to our reaching out to him in his comatose state, his case points out the importance of relating to unconscious people as if they can hear us even though we have no way of knowing whether we have made contact. I hope this report will stimulate others to reach out to coma victims – perhaps with the aid of sophisticated biofeedback devices to enable both parties to achieve contact.

CHAPTER 11
The doctor of the future

> The doctor of the future
> will give no medicine,
> but will interest his patients
> in the care of the human frame,
> in diet, and in the cause
> and prevention of disease.
>
> THOMAS A. EDISON
> 1847–1931

Third Line Medicine, in my view, is a young but vital new movement which provides contemporary medical practice with a much needed transfusion of ecologic and humanistic consciousness. It presses modern physicians to return to their Hippocratean roots, to avoid the beguiling simplicity of the doctrine of specific etiology, and to deal instead with the many interacting factors which influence our state of health. Most of all, it recognizes that the practice of medicine is an art which utilizes science, and calls for standards of practice which require not only knowledge, but also wisdom.

Despite its promise, however, Third Line medicine is no panacea. Even if it becomes generally accepted as a part of the health care system, it falls far short of solving the problems inherent in the current system. It is, after all, a participant in the process of compartmentalization upon which specialty medicine is based; its approach and procedures should not be tacked on at the end of the line, but should be integrated into all aspects of medical practice. It doesn't make sense for safer procedures to be used only when more dangerous procedures have failed to be effective. It doesn't make sense for patients to become alienated by high technology medicine only to re-establish a direct and caring relationship with physicians after high technology medicine has failed.

Third Line Medicine, while it improves the quality of medical care, is still only a stop-gap measure, still only a band-aid, until fundamental changes can be made in the modern system of medical practice. Medicine must abandon the doctrine of specific etiology and return to the ecologic model of Hippocrates. It must return to the principle of 'primum non nocere' (first do no harm), choosing safe procedures before dangerous ones, and learn to utilize the power of the placebo rather than to eliminate it. It must stop permitting machines to come between doctors and patients, and restore the physician-patient relationship to a central position in the delivery of health care services. Finally, it must return to treating patients as people, rather than as carriers of disease.

These changes should not be to the detriment of medicine's allegiance to science. Medical research should continue to be encouraged, and the results of scientific research should continue to influence the practice of medicine. I would like to see certain changes, however, in the manner in which research proposals are selected for funding. I would like to see preference given to interdisciplinary studies as it is these studies which build bridges between highly specialized and isolated areas of knowledge so as to prevent the distorted perceptions which scientists working with a narrow model are prone to develop.

I would also like to see preference given to studies which seek to determine the validity of controversial medical treatments. It is possible to prove whether or not such treatments are efficacious, even when the mechanism by which they work is undetermined. At the least, they can be compared to standard treatments. If they are proven ineffective, they should be abandoned; but if they are proven to be effective, they should be fostered. There is no good reason for any medical treatment to remain controversial for long.

One method by which this may be accomplished would be by the formation of committees of distinguished physicians which would review the scientific literature on each of the major controversial treatments to determine whether their safety and efficacy had been adequately investigated and, if not, to recommend specific studies which would permit conclusions to be reached. Each committee might consist of equal numbers of enthusiasts and skeptics along with a statistician who could both construct research protocols and evaluate protocols which would be submitted by others. Hopefully, funding sources would be willing to grant funds for such studies once the appropriate committee had concluded that a research proposal met its criteria for approval.

I should note that the British Medical Association has already taken the lead in this matter by forming a committee, the Working Party of Alternative Therapy, to consider ways of assessing the value of alternative therapies. In calling for information on alternative therapies, James Payne, the committee's chairman, has stated that: 'Our minds are open. Much success is being claimed for alternative therapy so we believe the time is right to gather information.' (*American Medical News* 9 September 1983) The committee is attempting to make a comprehensive assessment of the value of alternative medicine in helping patients and has been soliciting input from physicians, alternative therapists, and the public.

Lastly, I would like to see preference given to studies which investigate methods of fostering the process of self-healing. At the present time, most studies investigating the efficacy of a medical treatment compare the 'active' treatment with a placebo. It seems to me that it is equally important, or perhaps even more important, to fund studies which compare one form of placebo to another so as to discover how to intensify the processes by which we are capable of fostering healing within ourselves.

If medical practice is to become truly ecologic in scope, it must shift its concentration from the treatment of illness to the prolongation of health by the *prevention* of illness. With all that has been proven concerning the importance of poor personal habits in causing disease, how many first line physicians educate their healthy patients as to what lifestyle changes they could make in order to reduce their odds of future illness? Medicine today is all too passive in permitting illness to develop; only afterwards do physicians rush in and devote themselves to rescuing their patients from a process which they had ignored until it became manifest. John W. Farquhar, founder of the Stanford Heart Disease Prevention Program, warns that:

> the medical profession still hasn't really awakened to the fact that the concepts of health and prevention are changing. On one level, doctors' future economic livelihood is threatened unless they wake up. On another level, they've abdicated an important responsibility. (*Let's Live* February, 1982)

There are hopeful indications, however, that the doctor of the future will be wide awake. Medical education is changing, albeit slowly, and there is a growing trend to broaden the perspectives of future physicians as they pass through each phase of the educational process. Recently, for example, the AMA Council on Medical Education asked medical schools to endorse a liberal education in their admissions literature and otherwise act to reassure skeptical pre-med students that they are seeking applicants with a liberal arts background (Jenkins).

Even more encouraging is the recent 'revolt against Flexner' led by the Association of American Medical Colleges, the organization which represents all 127 medical schools in the United States as well as all sixteen medical schools in Canada. Steven Muller, President of Johns Hopkins University and chairman of a panel established by the AAMC to perform the first sweeping examination of American medical education since that of Flexner half a century ago, has stated that: 'We are doing an excellent job in training clinical scientists, but there are some things medical students are not getting, in part because of the extraordinary dosage of science they receive.' (Schwartz)

According to Muller, science is far more a method of inquiry than a body of facts; thus scientific aptitude lies more in the understanding and disciplined application of concepts than in the memorization of data (Hinz). John A. D. Cooper, President of the AAMC, agrees and adds that present medical education absorbs students 'so much that they don't have time to develop as human beings.' (op. cit.) Not only are these the views of Drs Muller and Cooper, but the results of a questionnaire distributed by the AAMC indicate that their views are shared by an overwhelming consensus of 1,000 medical school administrators, faculty and students (op. cit.).

In its report, issued in 1984, the panel made twenty-seven recommendations for medical education, including:

- an emphasis on broad-based education in the humanities and natural sciences
- modified admission requirement so that all qualified students – despite their majors – are considered seriously
- elevation of the status of teaching for instructors who often are hired and promoted on the basis of their research. (Hinz)

In medical school curricula, innovative programs are starting to appear which seek to broaden students' perspectives and to diminish the traditional splits. In Dallas, at the University of Texas Southwestern Medical School, a new program seeks to imbue enthusiasm for preventive medicine in its first year medical students. Students become objects of a study in preventive cardiology. Each is tested to assess individual risk factors for heart disease and is then given mental and physical stress tests to assess cardiovascular fitness. Each is asked to keep a diet diary and measures are taken to bring the risk factors under control. In addition, a seminar is tied to the experiential program which teaches such topics as stress management and nutrition (Mazer).

At the University of California School of Medicine, San Francisco, psychiatry has been incorporated into the medical clerkships of the third and fourth year students. Third year medical students traditionally tend to dehumanize their patients – but carefully documented attitude studies of the UC San Francisco students have shown a reversal of this trend (Jancin).

For medical school graduates, new residency programs are incorporating psychiatry into internal medicine to produce a new breed of specialist who is certified in both internal medicine and psychiatry. This integrated program was so successful at the West Virginia University School of Medicine that, when several faculty members moved to the University of Virginia School of Medicine, they quickly proceeded to develop a similar program there (Shemo *et al.*).

Progressive changes such as these are evidence that future physicians will have a broader perspective on the nature of illness. Yet, even if physicians return wholeheartedly to the ecologic model, ecologic medicine may continue to be hampered by a factor which no longer leaves the decision as to what occurs between physician and patient entirely in their hands. Because of the enormous cost of modern medical care, the major economic burden for medical services has shifted from the consumer to third party insurers, both private and governmental, which attempt to control costs by limiting the procedures for which they will approve payment. Thus, through the power of the pocketbook, impersonal insurance companies and Government agencies now exert a powerful influence upon the practice of medicine.

Medical insurance is one of the institutions which developed during the height of popularity of the doctrine of specific etiology. Both its analyses of medical services and its payment policies are predicated upon the tenets of specific etiology doctrine – and have yet to show major signs of progressive changes.

The current policies of third party carriers can be roughly translated into the following guidelines for physicians:

1 Physicians should sharply limit their verbal interactions with their patients and concentrate instead upon performing procedures and taking actions. (The more patients physicians see in an hour, and the more procedures they perform, the more they are paid.)
2 Surgery is the preferred method of treatment. (Physicians are paid vastly more for performing surgery than for any type of service – and there are no requirements for surgical procedures to be proven effective.)
3 Physicians should avoid treating the psychological aspects of their patients' illnesses. (Psychiatric services are frequently disallowed or reimbursed at a much lower level than are most other medical services.)
4 Physicians should only offer procedures which are generally accepted by the medical community. (Payment is usually disallowed for controversial procedures, even after all generally accepted procedures have failed.)
5 Physicians should not try to prevent illness. (Physicians' services are usually eligible for payment only when they are treating an established illness.)

Third party payers justify these policies by arguing that they are what the public wants. True, if the average healthy person today was asked to choose a health insurance plan based on such policies – and told that, the more the plan covered, the more it would cost – he or she would probably choose exactly the type of coverage which is commonly provided.

Suppose, however, that a plan were offered (either by the insurance industry or by the Government) which, instead of being based on specific etiology doctrine, was based on the principles of ecologic medicine. Physicians' services would be paid at an hourly rate determined by their amount of training and demonstrated expertise, not by the procedures they utilized. Preventive health care would be covered as would psychiatric services. Expensive procedures would only be covered it if could be justified that inexpensive procedures would be insufficient and, to encourage self-care, all subscribers would have to pay an initial fee for services.

Except for emergency situations, potentially dangerous procedures (like surgery) would only be covered if relatively safe procedures – first the proven ones and then the major unproven ones – had already been found to be ineffective. Even then, the unproven, dangerous procedures would be covered only if the proven ones had already been found to be ineffective.

We can only guess at what the cost of such a plan would be. If we base that guess on the evidence presented in this book, not only might it provide far better care, but it would probably cost substantially less than current insurance plans and socialized systems of medical care – and avert the growing health care crisis in western medicine which is placing the cost of medical services beyond the reach of the average consumer.

The only problem is that, for such a plan to work in countries where the delivery of medical services is not socialized, physicians must accept a radical restructuring in their charges. Unless the law of supply and demand would succeed in lowering surgical fees so that they are more in keeping with those charged for cognitive services, Government intervention may be necessary before the plan would be effective.

Although, in the United States, the current insurance picture is bleak, there are a few rays of light. Some carriers are beginning not only to accept charges for second opinions prior to surgery, but they are starting to demand it. The State of Massachusetts now has a law requiring that psychiatric services be included in all comprehensive plans for medical insurance. Finally, in 1982, Blue Shield of California announced that it would not pay for the latest 'breakthrough' in cardiac surgery (percutaneous transluminal coronary angioplasty) unless the doctor had performed it seventy-five times. Insurance experts say it is the first time that an insurance company has not routinely paid for an operation which has yet to be thoroughly evaluated (Nelson).

The doctrine of specific etiology fostered a model of the relationship between physicians and patients in which patients merely present themselves to their doctors who then proceed to diagnose and treat them. According to the model, the patient's responsibility is to comply with the doctor's orders. Ecologic medicine, on the other hand, is based on the establishment of a healing alliance between doctor and patient. The patient's responsibility is to become actively involved in the treatment process. This includes questioning and confronting the doctor as well as negotiating with him or her the nature of the treatment plan. In ecologic medicine, patients take responsibility for their health instead of leaving all the responsibility to their physicians.

Now that the era in which western medicine has been ruled by the doctrine of specific etiology is drawing to a close, the time has come for the public to assume the active role in health care which ecologic medicine envisions for it – both by demanding progressive changes in the economics of the multi-billion dollar health care industry and by demanding that their doctors respond to their needs by listening to them, by teaching them how to improve their state of health . . . and by showing them that they care.

APPENDIX

Third line physicians: how to find them

Third Line Medicine is a movement which, until now, has developed informally in response to a growing need from the public. Perhaps, now that this book has delineated this medical specialty, the time has come for third line physicians to develop a formal identity. Physicians interested in becoming involved in forming a professional society devoted to the development of Third Line Medicine are welcome to write to the author in care of the publisher; others seeking to support such a society are also welcome to write.

Until Third Line Medicine becomes organized, locating third line physicians will take some searching, especially because physicians whose medical practices fit my description of Third Line Medicine have yet to identify themselves with a unique label. The best place to begin is with your personal physicians. Describe Third Line Medicine to them (or better, suggest that they read this book) and ask them if they know of reputable colleagues whose background and interests approximate that description.

If your doctors have no suggestions, medical associations can give you leads. Many third line physicians belong to their national medical associations; however, these associations usually only categorize their members along traditional specialty lines. Contacting some of the smaller professional societies listed below for referral to local members will be more productive, since third line physicians constitute a significant portion of their membership.

These organizations can usually refer you to practicing physicians in your area who are knowledgeable about one or more of the treatments utilized by third line physicians, and they may be able to give you limited information regarding the nature of these physicians' medical practices. They cannot, however, tell you whether a physician practices Third Line

Medicine or comment upon his or her skills or reputation.

Thus, if you are referred to physicians through a professional society, you will still need to gather further information about them. Call their offices and ask about their training, experience, fees, and professional interests. Find out the range of diagnostic and therapeutic procedures which they utilize in their practices, and ask what they may have to offer to a person who has already seen appropriate medical specialists but is still unrelieved.

If you believe that you have found a physician who may be able to help you, do your final screening when you see the doctor for an evaluation. Evaluate the doctor just as he or she will be evaluating you; only then will you be able to decide if you have come to see the right person.

GENERAL INTERESTS:

International:

International Academy of Holistic Health and Medicine
218 Avenue B
Redondo Beach, California 90277
USA
(213) 540-0564

International Academy of Preventive Medicine
P.O. Box 25276
Shawnee Mission, Kansas 66225
USA
(913)631-3855

Canada:

Canadian Holistic Health Association
c/o Ted Leyton, MD
113 1/2 Lower Union Street
Kingston, Ontario K7L 2N3
(613) 542-5663

United Kingdom:

British Holistic Medical Association
179 Gloucester Place,
London NW1 6DX
England

Centre for the Study of Alternative Therapies
51 Bedford Place
Southampton, Hampshire SO1 2DG
England

England:
The McCarrison Society
President
Dr W. W. Yellowlees MB, ChB
Duiness
Aberfeldy, Perthshire PHIS 2ET
Scotland

United States of America:
American Holistic Medical Association
6932 Little River Turnpike
Annandale, Virginia 22003
(703) 642-5880

Northwest Academy of Preventive Medicine
15615 Bellevue – Redmond Road, Suite E
Bellevue, Washington 98008
(206) 881-9660

SPECIALIZED INTERESTS:

Acupuncture:

United Kingdom:
Association of Acupuncturists
238 Dyke Road
Brighton BN1 5AE
England

United States of America:
American Academy of Acupuncture Medicine
1504 North Madison
Anderson, Indiana 46012
(317) 642-2222

Center for Chinese Medicine
5266 East Pomona Boulevard
Los Angeles, California 90002
(213) 721-0774

Biofeedback Training:

Europe:
Paolo Pancheri, MD
European Biofeedback Society
Institute of Psychiatry
Viale de Universita 30
Rome, Italy

United States of America:
Biofeedback Society of America
10200 West 44th Avenue, #304
Wheat Ridge, Colorado 80033
(303) 420-2889

Clinical Ecology:

Canada:
Public Organizations:
Allergy Information Association
Room 7, 25 Poynter Drive
Weston, Ontario M9R 1K8

The Human Ecology Foundation of Canada
R.R. #1, Goodwood
Ontario LOC 1AO

United Kingdom:
Professional Society:
British Clinical Ecology Society
The Burgh Wood Clinic
34 Brighton Road
Banstead
Surrey SM7 1BS

Public Organization:
Action Against Allergy (AAA)
43 The Downs
London SW20 8HG
(01) 947-5082

United States of America:
Professional Society:
American Academy of Environmental Medicine
P.O. Box 16106
Denver, Colorado 80216
(303) 622-9755

Public Organization:
Human Ecology Action League (HEAL)
P.O. Box 1369
Evanston, Illinois 60204-1369

Nutritional Medicine:

International:
International College of Applied Nutrition
Box 386
La Habra, California 90631
USA

United Kingdom:
British Society for Nutritional Medicine
Membership Secretary and Treasurer
Dr Patrick Kingsley
MBBS, BA, D.Obst., RCOG
72 Main Street
Osgathorpe
Leicester LE12 9TA

Green Farm Nutrition Centre
Burnash Common
East Sussex TN19 7LA

Orthomolecular Treatment:

International:
Academy of Orthomolecular Psychiatry
1691 Northern Boulevard
Manhasset, New York 11030
USA
(516) 627-7535

Orthomolecular Medical Society
6551 W. Century Blvd., Suite 114
Los Angeles, California 90045
USA
(213) 417-7917

Pain Control:
International:
International Association for the Study of Pain
909 N.E. 43rd Street, Room 204
Seattle, Washington, 98105-6020
USA

Australia:
Australian Pain Society
c/o Dr D.A. Cherry
Dept. of Anaesthesia and Intensive Care
Flinders Medical Centre
Bedford Park, SA 5042

Canada:
Canadian Chapter
International Association for the Study of Pain
c/o Dr Barry Sessle
Faculty of Dentistry, University of Toronto
124 Edward Street
Toronto ON Canada M5G 1G6

New Zealand:
New Zealand Pain Society
c/o Dr Michael T.S. Roberts
24 Rewarewa Place
Matua
Tauranga, New Zealand

United Kingdom:
British and Irish Chapter
International Assoc. for the Study of Pain
c/o Dr Raymond G. Hill
Parke-Davis Research Unit
Addenbrookes Hospital Site
Hills Road
Cambridge CB2 England

United States of America:
American Pain Society
c/o Evelyne Hallberg
70 West Hubbard – Suite 202
Chicago, Illinois 60610
(312) 644-2623

Bibliography

CHAPTER 2

Bigelow, Joseph, *Brief Expositions of Rational Medicine*, Boston, Phillips, Sampson and Company, 1858.

Brown, E. Richard, *Rockefeller Medicine Men: Medicine and Capitalism in America*, Berkeley, California, University of California Press, 1979.

Coulter, Harris L., *Divided Legacy: A History of the Schism in Medical Thought*, Washington, DC, Wehawken Book Company, volume I, 1975.

Dubos, René, *Mirage of Health*, New York, Harper & Row, 1971.

Flexner, Abraham, *Medical Education in the United States and Canada, Bulletin no.* 4, New York, Carnegie Foundation for the Advancement of Teaching, 1910.

McKeown, Thomas, *The Role of Medicine: Dream, Mirage, or Nemesis*? Princeton, New Jersey, Princeton University Press, 1979.

CHAPTER 3

Arehart-Treichel, Joan, 'Life expectancy: The great 20th century leap', *Science News* 121: 186-8, 13 March 1982.

Avorn, J., Chen, M., Hartley, R., 'Scientific versus commercial sources of influence on the prescribing behavior of physicians', *American Journal of Medicine* 73:4, 1982.

Bechtel, Stefan, 'Medical tests: Don't bet your life on them'. *Prevention* January 1983, pp. 54-9.

Beecher, H.K., 'Surgery as a placebo', *Journal of the American Medical Association* 176:1102, 1961.

Bennett, Ivan L., Jr., 'Technology as a shaping force', in Knowles, John H., (ed.) *Doing Better and Feeling Worse: Health in the United States*, New York, W.W. Norton & Company, 1977.

Bradshaw, John S., *Doctors on Trial*, New York and London, Paddington Press Ltd., 1978, p. 31.

Bricklin, Mark, 'Journey to health: The right direction for a longer life', *Prevention*, September, 1980.

Brown, Sue, 'Your patients are turning up the heat', *Medical Economics*, 30 May 1983, pp. 130-6.

Bunker, J.P., Hinkley, D. and McDermott, W.V., 'Surgical innovation and its evaluation', *Science* 200: 937-41, 1978.

Butterworth, C.E., 'The skeleton in the hospital closet', *Nutrition Today* 9:4-8, 1974.

Chipponi, J. *et al.*, 'Total parenteral nutrition (TPN) often causes nutrient deficiences', *American Journal of Clinical Nutrition*, May 1982, pp. 1112-16.

Cook, Fred J. *The Plot Against the Patient*, Englewood Cliffs, New Jersey, Prentice-Hall, 1967.

Couch, N.P., Tilney, N.L., Rayner, A.A. and Moore, F.D., 'The high cost of low-frequency events: The anatomy and economics of surgical mishaps', *The New England Journal of Medicine* 304:634-7, 12, March 1981.

Daly and Hulka, 'Talking with the doctor (2)', *Journal of Communication*, Summer, 1978, p. 148.

Ehrlich, David Alan, *The Health-Care Cost Explosion: Which Way Now*? Bern, 1975, pp. 12-16, 22-3.

Epstein, Samuel, 'Cancer: Twisting the statistics about its causes', *Los Angeles Times*, 19 May 1981.

Evans, H.E., 'Tonsillectomy and adenoidectomy: Review of published evidence for and against T & A', *Clinical Pediatrics* 7:71-5, 1968.

Freese, Arthur S., *Managing your Doctor: How to Get the Best Possible Medical Care*, Briarcliff Manor, New York, Stein and Day, 1974.

Geller, Stephen, 'Autopsy', *Scientific American*, March, 1983.

Gilbert, J.P., McPeek, B. and Mosteller, F., 'Statistics and ethics in surgery and anesthesia', *Science*, 18 November 1977, pp. 684-9.

Goldman, L., Sayson, R., Robbins, S. *et al.*, 'The value of the autopsy in three medical eras', *The New England Journal of Medicine* 308:1000-5, 28 April 1983.

Heart Facts, Dallas, Texas, American Heart Association, 1985.

Hiatt, Howard H., 'Protecting the medical commons: Who is responsible?' *The New England Journal of Medicine* 293:235-41, 1975.

Hill, J.D., Hampton, J.R. and Mitchell, J.R.A., 'A randomized trial of home-versus-hospital management for patients with suspected myocardial infarction', *The Lancet* 1:837, 1978.

Holmberg, Scott D. and Faich, Gerald A., *Journal of the American Medical Association*, November, 1983.

House of Representatives, Committee on Interstate and Foreign Commerce, *Cost and Quality of Health Care: Unnecessary Surgery*,

Washington, D.C., US Government Printing Office, 1976.
Illich, Ivan, *Medical Nemesis*, New York, Random House, 1976.
Jacobs, Paul, 'Prescribing drugs: The hard sell', *Los Angeles Times* 29 December 1982.
Jick, Hershel, 'Drugs – remarkably nontoxic', *The New England Journal of Medicine* 291:824-8, 1974.
Kannel, William B., 'Meaning of the downward trend in cardiovascular mortality', *Journal of the American Medical Association*, 247:877-80, 1982.
Klevey, L.M., Reck, S.J. and Barcome, D.F., 'Evidence of dietary copper and zinc deficiencies', *Journal of the American Medical Association* 241:1916-18, 1979.
Knowles, John H., 'The responsibility of the individual', in Knowles, John H., (ed.) *Doing Better and Feeling Worse: Health in the United States*, New York, W.W. Norton & Company, 1977.
Krehl, Williard A., 'The evaluation of nutritional status', *The Medical Clinics of North America* 48:1129-40, 1964.
Lander, Louise, *Defective Medicine: Risk, Anger and the Malpractice Crisis*, New York, Farrar, Straus and Giroux, 1978.
Lemoine A., Le Devehat, C., Codaccioni J.L. *et al.*, 'Vitamin B1, B2, B6, and C status in hospital inpatients', *The American Journal of Clinical Nutrition* 33: 2595-260, 1980.
Mather, H.G., Pearson, W.G., Read, K.L.Q. *et al.*, 'Acute myocardial infarction, home and hospital treatment', *British Medical Journal* 3:334-8, 1971.
Mayer, Jean quoted in Cheraskin, E. and Ringsdorf, W.M., *Predictive Medicine*, New Canaan Connecticut, Keats Publishing Company, 1977.
McKeown, Thomas, *The Role of Medicine: Dream, Mirage, or Nemesis*? Princeton, New Jersey, Princeton University Press, 1979.
McKinley, James, 'The pusher in the gray-flannel suit', *Playboy* 25: 165(7), September 1978.
Morgan, John P. quoted in 'Prescribing: A broader perspective', *Drug Therapy*, December, 1981.
Mullen, J.L., Buzby, G.P., Matthews, D.C. *et al.*, 'Reduction of operative morbidity and mortality by combined preoperative and postoperative nutritional support', *Annals of Surgery* 192:604-13, 1980.
Paradise, J.L., 'Why T & A remains moot', *Pediatrics* 49: 648-51, 1972.
Preston, Thomas A., 'Bypass surgery: A placebo?', *MD* February, 1985, pp. 30-8.
Rudman, Daniel, 'Protein-energy undernutrition', in Isselbacher, Kurt J., Adams, Raymond D., Braunwald, Eugene, *et al.*, (eds)

Harrison's Principles of Internal Medicine, New York, McGraw-Hill, 1980.

Rynearson, Robert R., 'Touching people', *Journal of Clinical Psychiatry* 39-492, June, 1978.

Siebert, W.H., *Proceedings of the First Conference on Electronics in Medicine*, New York, McGraw-Hill, 1969.

Snyder, Paul, *Health and Human Nature*, Radnor, Pennsylvania, Chilton Book Company, 1980, p. 74.

Stamler, J., 'Primary prevention of coronary heart disease: The last 20 years', *American Journal of Cardiology* 47:722-35, 1981.

Steffee, William P., 'Malnutrition in hospitalized patients', *Journal of the American Medical Association* 244:2630-5, 1980.

Talley, Robert B. and Laventurier, Marc F., 'Drug-induced illness', *Journal of the American Medical Association* 229:1043, 1974.

Thomas, Lewis, *The Lives of a Cell: Notes of a Biology Watcher*, New York, The Viking Press, 1974.

Thomas, Lewis, 'On the science and technology of medicine', in Knowles, John H., (ed.) *Doing Better and Feeling Worse: Health in the United States*. New York, W.W. Norton, 1977.

Thomas, Lewis, *The Medusa and the Snail: More Notes of a Biology Watcher*, New York, The Viking Press, 1979.

Thompson, J.S., Burrough, C.A., Green, J.L. and Brown, G.L., 'Nutritional screening in surgical patients', *Journal of the American Dietetic Association* 84(3):337-8, 1984.

Tomasson, Richard F., 'The mortality of Swedish and U.S. white males: A comparison of experience, 1969-1971', *The American Journal of Public Health* 66:968-74, 1976.

Trafford, Abigail, 'America's $39 billion heart business', *U.S. News and World Report*, 15 March 1982.

Trubo, Richard, 'The Achilles' heel of medicine', *Medical World News* January 1985, pp. 127-35.

Truent, P., Le Gall, J., Lhoste, F. *et al.*, 'The role of iatrogenic disease in admissions to intensive care', *Journal of the American Medical Association* 244:2617-20, 12 December 1980.

White, Jane See, 'Opinion surveys: You're not doing as well as you think', *Medical Economics* 27 June 1983, pp. 67-8.

Wildavsky, Aaron, 'Doing better and feeling worse: The political pathology of health pathology', in Knowles, John H., (ed.) *Doing Better and Feeling Worse: Health in the United States*, New York, W.W. Norton, 1977.

Williams, Roger J., *Nutrition Against Disease*, New York, Pitman Publishing Company, 1971.

Wright, Richard A., 'Nutritional assessment', *Journal of the American Medical Association* 244:559-60, 1980.

Zucker, Martin, 'Americans, change your eating habits!' *Let's Live*, September, 1982.

CHAPTER 4

Almy, T.P., 'The role of the primary physician in the healthcare industry', *The New England Journal of Medicine* 304:225, 1981.

Brown, A.C. and Fry, J., 'The Cornell Medical Index Health Questionnaire in the identification of neurotic patients in general practice', *Journal of Psychosomatic Research* 6:185-90, 1962.

Cannon, Walter B., *Bodily Changes in Pain, Hunger, Fear and Rage*, New York, Appleton, 1929.

Chase, Robert A., 'Proliferation of certification in medical specialties: Productive or counter-productive', *The New England of Medicine* 294:497-9, 1976.

Cooper, B. and Sylph, J., 'Life events and the onset of neurotic illness: An investigation in general practice', *Psychological Medicine* 3:421-35, 1973.

Fink, Paul J., 'Psychiatry must remain a medical specialty', in Brady, John Paul and Brodie, H. Keith, (eds) *Controversies in Psychiatry*, Philadelphia, W.B. Saunders, 1978.

Hall, R.C.W., Gardner, E.R., Stickney, S.K. *et al.*, 'Physical illness manifesting as psychiatric disease', *Archives of General Psychiatry* 37:989-95, 1980.

Hall, R.C.W., Popkin, M.K., DeVaul, R.A. *et al.*, 'Physical illness presenting as psychiatric disease', *Archives of General Psychiatry* 35:1315-20, 1978.

Holverson, Harmon E., 'Family practice is becoming the first victim of competition', *Medical Economics* 4 February 1985, pp. 29-33.

Johnson, D.A.W., 'The evaluation of routine physical examination in psychiatric cases', *Practitioner* 200:686-91, 1968.

Jones, D.R. and Vischi, T.R., 'Impact of alcohol, drug abuse, and mental health treatment on medical care utilization: a review of the research literature', *Medical Care* 17:12, 1979.

Kaplan, Harold I., 'Psychophysiological disorders', in Freedman, A.F., Kaplan, H.I. and Sadock, B.J., (eds) *Comprehensive Textbook of Psychiatry III*, Baltimore, The Williams & Wilkins Company, 1980.

Koiton, W., Ries, R.K., Kleinman, A., 'The prevalence of somatization in primary care', *Comprehensive Psychiatry* 25:208-215, 1984.

Koranyni, Erwin K., 'Somatic illness in psychiatric patients', *Psychosomatics* 21:887-91, 1980.

Levit, Edithe J., Sabshin, Melvin and Mueller, Barber, C., 'Trends in graduate medical education and specialty certification', *The New*

England Journal of Medicine 290:545-9, 7 March 1974.

Lipowski, Z.J., 'Consultation-liaison psychiatry: An overview', *The American Journal of Psychiatry* 131:623-30, June, 1974.

McIntyre, S. and Romano, J., 'Is there a stethoscope in the house (and is it used)?' *Archives of general Psychiatry*34:1147-51, 1975.

Nielsen, Arthur C., III, 'Psychiatric recruitment: Why they like us, but don't join us', *Psychosomatics* 22:343-8, April 1981.

Parloff, M.B., 'Can psychotherapy research guide the policymaker? A little knowledge may be a dangerous thing', *American Psychologist* 34:296-306, 1979.

Paulshock, Bernadine Z., 'Why specialists are stealing more patients than ever', *Medical Economics* 26 December 1983, pp. 25-6.

A Psychiatric Glossary, fifth edn, Washington DC, American Psychiatric Association, 1980.

Rosen, George, *The Specialization of Medicine*, New York, Froben Press, 1944.

Schlesinger, H.J., Mumford, E., Glass, G.V. *et al.*, 'Mental health utilization in a fee-for-service system: Outpatient mental health treatment following the onset of a chronic disease', *American Journal of Public Health* 73:422-9, 1983.

Singer, Charles and Underwood, E. Ashworth, *A Short History of Medicine*, second edition, London, Oxford University Press, 1962.

Stacey, James, 'Controversy continues to surround psychiatry', *American Medical News*, 16 June 1982.

Stollerman, Gene H., 'The gold standard', *Hospital Practice* 30 January 1985.

Wassersug, Joseph D., 'Subspecialists are squeezing me out', *Medical Economics* 18, February 1985, p. 65.

Wechsler, H., Dorsey, J.L. and Bovey, J.D., 'A follow-up study of residents in internal medicine, pediatrics and obstetrics-gynecology training programs in Massachusetts', *The New England Journal of Medicine* 298:15-21, 5 January 1978.

CHAPTER 5

Abercrombie, John, *Inquiries Concerning the Intellectual Powers and the Investigation of Truth*, New York, Harper and Brothers, 1834, p. 297.

Brownell, Kelly D. and Stunkard, Albert J., 'The double-blind in danger: Untoward consequences of informed consent', *American Journal of Psychiatry* 139:1487-9, 1982.

Byington, Robert P. *et al.*, (eds) *Journal of the American Medical Association*, 22/29 March 1985.

Capra, Fritjof, 'Zen and subatomic physics', *New Society*, 20 November 1975.

Cohen, Morris R. and Nagel, Ernest, *An Introduction to Logic and the Scientific Method*, New York, Harcourt Brace Jovanovitch 1934, pp. 382-3.

Dubos, René, *Mirage of Health*, New York, Harper & Row, 1971.

Einstein, Albert and Infeld, Leopold, *The Evolution of Physics*, New York, Simon & Shuster, 1942.

Feinstein, Alvan R., Horwitz, Ralph I., Spitzer, Walter O. and Battista, Renaldo N., 'Coffee and pancreatic cancer: The problems of etiologic science and epidemiologic case-control research', *The Journal of the American Medical Association* 246:957-61, 28 August 1981.

Fries, James. 'Aging, natural death, and the compression of morbidity', *The New England Journal of Medicine* 303:130-5, 17 July 1980.

Hayek, F.A. 'The theory of complex phenomena', in *Studies of Philosophy, Politics and Economics*, Chicago, University of Chicago Press, 1967.

Hine, F.R., Werman, D.S. and Simpson, D.M., 'Effectiveness of psychotherapy: Problems of research on complex phenomena', *American Journal of Psychiatry* 139:204-8, February, 1982.

Kuhn, Thomas S., *The Structure of Scientific Revolutions*, Chicago, University of Chicago Press, 1970.

Lastrucci, Carol L., *The Scientific Approach: Basic Principles of the Scientific Method*, Cambridge, Massachusetts, Schenkman Publishing Company, 1963.

LeMaitre, George D., *How to Choose a Good Doctor*, Andover, Massachusetts, Andover Publishing Group, 1979.

McKeown, Thomas, *The Role of Medicine: Dream, Mirage, or Nemesis*? Princeton, New Jersey, Princeton University Press, 1979.

Morowitz, Harold J., 'Rediscovering the mind', *Psychology Today*, August, 1980.

Office of Technology Assessment, US Congress, 'Assessing the efficacy and safety of medical technology', US Government Printing Office, 1978, p. 7.

Osler, Sir William, *Aequanimitas and Other Addresses*, third edn, Philadelphia, The Blakiston Company, 1932.

Shipman, William G., Greene, Charles S., Laskin, Daniel M., 'Correlation of placebo responses and personality characteristics in myofascial pain-dysfunction (MPD) patients', *Journal of Psychosomatic Research* 18:475-83, 1974.

Williams, Roger J., *Physicians' Handbook of Nutritional Science*, Springfield, Illinois, Charles C. Thomas, 1975.

CHAPTER 6

Bahnson, Claus Bahne, 'Stress and cancer: The state of the art', *Psychosomatics* 21:975-81, 1980.

Bartrop, R.W., Lazurus, L., Luckhurst, E. *et al.*, 'Depressed lymphocyte function after bereavement', *The Lancet* 1:834-6, 1977.

Beecher, Henry K., *Measurement of Subjective Responses: Quantitative Effects of Drugs*, London, Oxford University Press, 1959.

Benson, Herbert, *The Relaxation Response*, New York, William Morrow and Company, 1975.

Benson, Herbert, Beary, John F. and Carol, Mark P., 'The relaxation response', *Psychiatry* 37:46, 1974.

Bergin, A.E. and Lambert, M.J., 'The evaluation of therapeutic outcomes' in Bergin, A.E. and Garfield, S.L., (ed) *Handbook of Psychotherapy and Behavior Change: An Empirical Analysis*, second edn, New York, John Wiley & Sons, 1978, pp. 138-9.

Berkman, L.F. and Syme, S.L., 'Social networks, host resistance, and mortality: A nine-year follow-up study of Alameda County residents', *American Journal of Epidemiology* 109: 186-204, 1979.

Brown, Barbara B., *Super-Mind: The Ultimate Energy*, New York, Harper & Row, 1980.

Buchsbaum, Monte S., 'The sensoristat in the brain', *Psychology Today*, May 1978, pp. 96-104.

Cassell, Eric, *The Healer's Art: A New Approach to the Doctor-Patient Relationship*, New York, J.P. Lippincott, 1976.

Cousins, Norman, 'The mysterious placebo: How mind helps medicine work', *The Saturday Review*, 1 October 1977, pp. 8-12.

Engel, George L., 'The need for a new medical model: A challenge for biomedicine', *Science* 196:129-36, 8 April 1977.

Engel, George L., 'The clinical application of the biopsychosocial model', *American Journal of Psychiatry* 137:535-44, May, 1980.

Evans, Frederick J., 'The power of a sugar pill', *Psychology Today*, April, 1974.

Frank, Jerome D., 'Therapeutic factors in psychotherapy', *American Journal of Psychotherapy* 25:350-61, 1971.

Friedman, M. and Rosenman, R.H., *Type A Behavior and Your Heart*, New York, Alfred A. Knopf, 1974.

Fryer, Barbara, 'Stress', *Los Angeles*, April, 1980.

Gatchel, Robert J. and Price, Kenneth P., (eds) *Clinical Applications of Biofeedback: Appraisal and Status*, New York, Pergamon Press, 1979.

Gold, H. in *Cornell Conferences on Therapy*, volume 1, edited by Gold, H. *et al.*, New York, Macmillan, 1946.

Holmes, Thomas H. and Masuda, Minoru, 'Psychosomatic syndrome',

Psychology Today, April, 1972.

Holmes, Thomas H. and Rahe, Richard H., 'The social readjustment scale', *Journal of Psychosomatic Research* 11:213-18, 1967.

Kielholz, P., (ed.) *Masked Depression*, Bern, Hans Huber, 1973.

Kleinman, Arthur M., 'Why do indigenous practitioners successfully heal?' *Proceedings of the Medical Anthropology Workshop on The Healing Process*, Michigan State University, 7-10 April 1976.

Kleinman, Arthur M. Eisenberg, Leon and Good, Byron, 'Culture, illness and care: Clinical lessons from anthropologic and cross-cultural research', *Annals of Internal Medicine* 88:251-8, 1978.

Knowles, John H., 'The responsibility of the individual' in Knowles, John H., (ed.) *Doing Better and Feeling Worse: Health in the United States*, New York, W.W. Norton, 1977.

Korneva, E.A., 'The effect of stimulating different mesencephalic structures on protective immune response pattern', *Fiziologiceskii zhurnal SSSR IM. I.M. Sechenova* 53:42, 1967.

La Barba, Richard C., 'Experimental and environmental factors in cancer: A review of research with animals', *Psychosomatic Medicine* 32:259-76, 1970.

Lattime, E.C. and Strausser, H.R., 'Arteriosclerosis: Is stress-induced immune supression a risk factor?' *Science* 198:302-3, 1977.

Leff, David N. 'Stress-triggered organic disease in this year of economic anxiety', *Medical World News*, 24 March 1975.

Lesse, Stanley, (ed.) *Masked Depression*, New York, Jason Aronson, 1974.

Levine, Jon D., Gordon, Newton C. and Fields, Howard L., 'The mechanism of placebo analgesia', *The Lancet* 2:654-7, 23 September 1978.

Lipowski, Z.J., 'Psychosomatic medicine in the seventies: An overview', *American Journal of Psychiatry* 134:233-44, 1977.

Miller, Neal, 'Learning of visceral and glandular responses', *Science* 163:434-45, 1969.

Moertel, C.G., Taylor, W.F., Roth, A. and Tyce, F.A.J., 'Who responds to sugar pills?' *Mayo Clinic Proceedings* 51:96-100, 1976.

Monjan, A.A. and Collector, M.I., 'Stress-induced modulation of the immune response', *Science* 196:307-8, 1977.

Nemiah, John C., 'Alexithymia and psychosomatic illness', *J.C.E. Psychiatry*, October, 1978, pp. 25-37.

Nerem, R.M., Levesque, M.J. *et al.*, 'Social environment as a factor in diet-induced atherosclerosis', *Science* 208:1475-6, June, 1980.

Park, L.C. and Covi, L., 'Non-blind placebo trial: An exploration of neurotic patients' responses to placebo when its inert content is disclosed'. *Archives of General Psychiatry* 12:336-45, 1965.

Peek, C.J., 'A critical look at the theory of placebo', *Biofeedback and*

Self-Regulation 2:327-35, 1977.

Peterson, E.A. Augenstein, J.S., Tanis, D.C. *et al.*, 'Noise raises blood pressure without impairing auditory sensitivity', *Science* 211:1450-2, 27 March 1981.

Petrie, Asenath, *Individuality in Pain and Suffering*, Chicago University of Chicago Press, 1967.

Riley, Vernon, 'Mouse mammary tumors: Alternation of incidence as apparent function of stress', *Science* 189:465-7, 1975.

Seligman, Martin E.P., 'Fall into helplessness', *Psychology Today*, June, 1973.

Shapiro, Arthur K., 'The placebo effect of treatment', *Drug Therapy*, December, 1971, pp. 45-54.

Shipman, William G., Greene, Charles S. and Laskin, Daniel L., 'Correlation of placebo responses and personality characteristics in myofascial pain-dysfunction (MPD) patients', *Journal of Psychosomatic Research* 18:475-83, 1974.

Sifneos, Peter, *Short-Term Psychotherapy and Emotional Crisis*, Cambridge, Massachusetts, Harvard University Press, 1972.

Silver, Bernard V. and Blanchard, Edward B., 'Biofeedback and relaxation training in the treatment of psychophysiological disorders: Or are the machines really necessary?' *Journal of Behavioral Medicine* 1:217-39, 1978.

Silverman, Samuel, *Psychologic Clues to Forecasting Physical Illness*, New York, Appleton-Centry-Crofts, 1970.

Simonton, O. Carl, Matthews-Simonton, Stephanie and Sparks, T. Flint, 'Psychological intervention in the treatment of cancer', *Psychosomatics* 21:226-33, 1980.

Skinner, James E., 'Heart-attack trigger', *Psychology Today*, July, 1980.

Sklar, Lawrence and Anisman, Hymie, 'Stress and coping factors influence tumor growth', *Science* 205:513-15, 3 August 1979.

Sternbach, R. and Tursky, B., 'Ethnic differences among housewives in psycho-physical and skin potential response to electric shock', *Psychophysiology* 1:241-6, 1965.

Stimson, G., 'Obeying doctor's orders', *Soc. Sci. Med.* 8:97-104, 1974.

Stoeckle, J. Zola, I.K. and Davidson, G., 'The quantity and significance of psychological distress in medical patients', *Journal of Chronic Diseases* 17:959-70, 1964.

Strupp, Hans H. and Hadley, Suzanne W. 'Specific vs. nonspecific factors in psychotherapy: A controlled study of outcome', *Archives of General Psychiatry* 36:1125-36, 1979.

Swisher, Scott N., 'The biopsychosocial model: Its future for the internist', *Psychosomatic Medicine* 42:113-21, 1980.

Totman, Richard, *Social Causes of Illness*, New York, Pantheon Books, 1979.

Truax, Charles B. and Carkhuff, Robert R., *Towards Effective Counseling and Psychotherapy: Training and Practice*, Chicago, Aldine Publishing Company, 1967.

Vaillant, George E., 'Natural history of male psychological health', *The New England Journal of Medicine* 301:1249-54, 1979.

Voss, Tom, 'Good friends and good health go hand in hand', *Prevention*, March 1981.

Weiss, Robert J., 'The biopsychosocial model and primary care', *Psychosomatic Medicine* 42:123-30, 1980.

Wickramasekera, Ian, 'A conditioned response model of the placebo effect: Predictions from the model', *Biofeedback and Self-Regulation* 5:5-18, 1980.

Zola, I.K., 'Culture and symptoms: An analysis of patients' presenting complaints.' *American Sociological Review* 615-30, 1966.

CHAPTER 7

Auersbacher, Anna, 'Aerobic exercise best bet to boost HDL levels', *Medical Tribune* 23 December 1981.

'Avoidable risks of cancer in the United States today', in *Assessment of Technologies for Determining Cancer Risks in the Environment*, Washington, DC, Office of Technology Assessment, 1981.

Belloc, N.B. and Breslow, L., 'Relationship of health practices and mortality', *Preventive Medicine* 2:57-81, 1973.

Boyd, W.d. Graham-White, J., Blackwood, G. *et al.*, 'Clinical effects of choline in Alzheimer senile dementia', *The Lancet* 2:711, 1977.

Brody, Jerome S., 'Tobacco smolders on', *The New England Journal of Medicine*, 298:48-9, 5 January 1978.

Burton, B.T., (Executive ed.) *The Heinz Handbook of Nutrition: A Comprehensive Treatise on Nutrition in Health and Disease*, New York, McGraw-Hill, 1959.

Cheraskin, E. and Ringdorf, W.M., Jr, 'Predictive medicine: V. Linear versus curvilinear functions', *Journal of the American Geriatrics Society* 19:721-8, August, 1971.

Frederick, Larry, 'Labeling cigarettes for what they are', *Medical World News*, 15 March 1982.

Friedmann, Lawrence W., 'Causes and treatment of low back pain', *Medical Tribune* 8 May 1974.

Gelenberg, A.J., Wojcik, J.D., Growdon, J.H. *et al.*, 'Tyrosine for the treatment of depression', *American Journal of Psychiatry* 137:622-3, May, 1980.

Ghadirian, A.M., Anath, J. and Englesmann, F., 'Folic acid deficiency and depression', *Psychosomatics* 21:926-9, November, 1980.

Griest, John H., Klein, Marjorie H., Eischens, Roger R. and Faris, John W., 'Antidepressant running', *Behavioral Medicine* June, 1978.

The Health Consequences of Smoking, Public Health Services Publication no. 1696, US Department of Health, Education and Welfare, 1967.

Hartmann, Ernest, 'L-tryptophan: A rational hypnotic with clinical potential', *American Journal of Psychiatry* 134:366-70, April, 1977.

Horwitz, Nathan, 'Diet can cut Ca risk; Question is how much', *Medical World News* 14 July 1982.

Knowles, John H., 'The responsibility of the individual' in Knowles, John H. (ed.) *Doing Better and Feeling Worse: Health in the United States*, New York, W.W. Norton & Company, 1977.

Kroger, William S., 'Acupuncture analgesia: Its explanation by conditioning theory, autogenic training and hypnosis', *American Journal of Psychiatry* 130:855-60, 1973.

Lee, Do Chil, Lee, Myung O. and Clifford, Donald H., 'Modification of cardiovascular function in dogs by acupuncture: A review', *American Journal of Chinese Medicine* 4:333-46, 1976.

Marmot, M. and Winkelstein, W., 'Epidemiologic observations on intervention trials for prevention of coronary heart disease', *American Journal of Epidemiology* 101:1277, 1975.

McKeown, Thomas, *The Role of Medicine: Dream, Mirage, or Nemesis?* Princeton, New Jersey, Princeton University Press, 1979.

Melzack, Ronald, Stillwell, Dorothy M. and Fox, Elisabeth J., 'Trigger points and acupuncture points for pain: correlations and implications', *Pain* 3:3-23, 1977.

Moskow, H.A. *et al.*, 'Alcohol, sludge, and hypoxic areas of nervous system, liver and heart', *Microvascular Research* 1:174, 1968.

National Academy of Sciences, *Recommended Dietary Allowances*, Washington, DC, US Government Printing Office, 1980.

Nockels, Cheryl F., 'Protective effects of supplemental vitamin E against infection', *Federation Proceedings* 38:377-94, 1975.

O'Connor, John and Bensky, Dan, (trans. and eds) 'A summary of research concerning the effects of acupuncture', Section from the book *Acupuncture* by the Shanghai College of Traditional Medicine, *American Journal of Chinese Medicine* 3:377-94, 1975.

Oleson, Terrence D., Kroening, Richard J. and Bresler, David E., 'An experimental evaluation of auricular diagnosis: The somatotopic mapping of musculoskeletal pain at ear acupuncture points', *Pain* 8:217-29, 1980.

Omura, Yoshiaki, 'Patho-physiology of acupuncture treatment: Effects of acupuncture on cardiovascular and nervous systems', *Acupuncture & Electro-Therapeutic Research* 1:51-140, 1975.

Paffenbarger, Ralph S. and Hyde, Robert T., 'Exercise as protection against heart attack', *The New England Journal of Medicine* 302:1026-7, 1 May 1980.

Pauling, Linus, 'On the orthomolecular environment of the mind: Orthomolecular theory', *American Journal of Psychiatry* 131:1251-7, November, 1974.

Pelletier, Omer, 'Vitamin C and cigarette smokers', *Annals of the New York Academy of Sciences* 258: 156-68, 1975.

Rao, B. and Broadhurst, A.D., 'Tryptophane and depression', *British Medical Journal* 1:460, 1976.

Riddle, Jackson W., (chair.) 'Report of the New York State Commission on acupuncture', *American Journal of Chinese Medicine* 2:289-318, 1974.

Rosenberg, L., Shapiro, S., Slone, D. *et al.*, 'Breast cancer and alcoholic-beverage consumption', *The Lancet* 30 January 1982, pp. 267-70.

Scala, James, *Nutrition Today*, September-October, 1980.

1982 *Surgeon General's Report on the Nation's Health*, Washington, DC, US Government Printing Office, 1982.

Task Force Report 7: Megavitamin and Orthomolecular Therapy in Psychiatry, Washington, DC, American Psychiatric Association, 1973.

Travell, J. and Rinzler, S.H., 'The myofascial genesis of pain'. *Postgraduate Medicine* 11:425-34, 1952.

United States Census Bureau, *Statistical Abstract of the United States*, 102nd annual edition, Washington, DC, US Government Printing Office, 1982.

Williams, Roger J., *Nutrition Against Disease*, New York, Pitman Publishing Company, 1971.

Williams, R.S., Logue, E.E., Lewis, J.L. *et al.*, 'Physical conditioning augments the fibrinolytic response to venous occlusion in healthy adults', *The New England Journal of Medicine* 302:987-91, 1980.

Winston, Mary, 'Diet and coronary heart disease', *Contemporary Nutrition* September, 1981.

Wright, Jonathan V., 'Expectations, reasonable and unreasonable', *Prevention* August, 1981, pp. 65-8.

Yates, John, 'A natural approach to Diabetes', *Prevention* January, 1981.

Yew, Man-Li, 'Recommended daily allowances for vitamin C', *Proceedings of the National Academy of Sciences* 70:969-72, April, 1973.

Zook, Christopher J. and Moore, Francis D., 'High-cost users of medical care', *The New England Journal of Medicine* 302:996-1002, 1 May 1980.

CHAPTER 8

Abram, Harry S., 'The psychology of chronic illness', *Annals, American Academy of Political and Social Science*, January, 1980.

Abroms, Gene A., 'The new eclecticism', *Archives of General Psychiatry* 20:514-23, 1969.

Ader, Robert, (ed.) *Psychoneuroimmunology*, New York, Academic Press, 1981.

Alexander, F.A.D., 'The control of pain', in Hale, D., (ed.) *Anesthesiology*, Philadelphia, F.A. Davis, 1954.

Angyal, Andras, *Neurosis and Treatment: A Holistic Theory*, New York, John Wiley & Sons, 1965.

Blackwell, Barry, 'Biofeedback in a comprehensive behavioral medicine program', *Biofeedback and Self-Regulation* 6:445-72, 1981.

Bonica, John J., 'General clinical considerations (including organization and function of a pain clinic)' in Bonica, John J., Procacci, Paolo and Pagni, Carlo A., (eds) *Recent Advances in Pain: Pathophysiology and Clinical Aspects*, Springfield, Illinois, Charles C. Thomas, 1974.

Kellner, Robert, 'Psychotherapy in psychosomatic disorders: A survey of controlled studies', *Archives of General Psychiatry* 32:1021-8, 1975.

Lipowski, Z.J., 'Consultation-liaison psychiatry: An overview', *The American Journal of Psychiatry* 131:623-30, 1974.

Meir, A., 'General systems theory', *Archives of General Psychiatry* 21:302-10, 1969.

Nelson, Harry, 'New holistic medicine: The spirit grows', *The Los Angeles Times* 25 December 1977.

Price, Kenneth P. 'The application of behavior therapy to the treatment of psychosomatic disorders: Retrospect and prospect', *Psychotherapy: Theory, Research and Practice* 11:138-55, Summer, 1974.

Relman, Arnold S., 'Holistic medicine', *The New England Journal of Medicine* 300:312-13, 8 February 1979.

Salminen, J.K., Lehtinen, V., Jokinen, K. *et al.*, 'Psychosomatic disorder: A treatment problem more difficult than neurosis?' *Acta Psychiatrica Scandinavia* 62:1-12, July, 1980.

Schwartz, Gary D. and Weiss, Stephen M., 'Behavioral medicine revisited: An amended definition', *Journal of Behavioral Medicine* 1:249-51, 1978.

Shealy, C. Norman, 'Holism, science and mysticism or how scientific is medicine?' *Journal of Holistic Medicine* 3:30-7, 1981.

Simon, Robert M., 'On eclecticism', *American Journal of Psychiatry* 131:135-9, 1974.

Stevens, Anita, 'The role of psychotherapy in psychosomatic disorders', *Behavioral Neuropsychiatry* 4:2-5, 1972.

CHAPTER 9

Abbey, Laraine C., 'Agoraphobia', *Journal of Orthomolecular Psychiatry* 11:243-59, 1982.

Axelrod. A.E., 'Immune processes in vitamin deficiency states', *American Journal of Clinical Nutrition* 24:265, 1971.

Boris, M., Shiff, M., Weindorf, S. and Inselman, I., 'Bronchoprovocation blocked by neutralization therapy', *Allergy and Clinical Immunology* 71:92 (supplement), 1983.

Brin, Myron, 'Drugs and environmental chemicals in relation to vitamin needs' in Hathcock, J.N. and Coon, J. (eds) *Nutrition and Drug Interrelationships*, New York, Academic Press, 1978, pp. 131-50.

Brin, Myron, 'Example of behavioral changes in marginal vitamin deficiency in the rat and man' in *Behavioral Effects of Energy and Protein Deficits*, Washington, DC, US, Department of Health, Education and Welfare (NIH Publication no. 79-1906), 1979.

Brin, Myron, 'Editorial: Red cell transketolase as an indicator of nutritional deficiency', *The American Journal of Clinical Nutrition* 33:169-71, 1980.

Brozek, J., 'Physiological effects of thiamine restriction and deprivation in young men', *American Journal of Clinical Nutrition* 5:109-120, 1957.

Crook, William G., *The Yeast Connection: A Medical Breakthrough*, second edn, Jackson, Tennessee, Professional Books, 1983 (available through Professional Books, P.O. Box 3494, Jackson, Tennessee 38301).

Cunningham-Rubdles, Charlotte *et al.*, 'Milk precipitins, circulating immune complexes and IgA deficiency', *Proceedings of the National Academy of Sciences* volume 75, number 7, July 1978.

Dohan, F.C. and Grasberger, J.C., 'Relapsed schizophrenics: Earlier discharge from the hospital after cereal-free, milk-free diet', *American Journal of Psychiatry* 130:685-8, 1973.

Domschke, W., Dichschas, A. and Mitznegg, P., 'CSF B-endorphin in schizophrenia', *The Lancet*, 12 May 1979, p. 1024.

'Efamol' Technical Information Bulletins. Efamol Research, Incorporated, P.O. Box 818, Kentville, Nova Scotia, Canada B4N 4H8.

Egger, J., Wilson, J., Carter, C.M., Turner, M.W. and Soothill, J.F., 'Is migraine food allergy?' *The Lancet* 15 October 1983, pp. 865-9.

Egger, J., Graham, P.J., Carter, C.M., Gumley, D. and Soothill, J.F.,

'Controlled trial of oligoantigenic treatment in the hyperkinetic syndrome', *The Lancet* 9 March 1985, pp. 540-5.

Finn, Ronald and Cohen, H. Newman, ' "Food allergy": Fact or fiction?' *The Lancet*, 25 February 1978, pp. 426-8.

Gay, D.D., Cox, R.D. and Reinhard, J.W., 'Chewing releases mercury from fillings'. *The Lancet* 5 May 1979, p. 985

Hanson, Mats, 'Amalgam – Hazards in your teeth', *Journal of Orthomolecular Psychiatry* 12:194-201, 1983.

Hodges, R.E., Baker, E.M., Hood, J. *et al.*, 'Experimental scurvy in man', *American Journal of Clinical Nutrition* 22:535-48, 1969.

Horiguti, Sinsak, 'The removal of the disorders of the autonomic nervous system', *Acupuncture & Electro-Therapeutic Research* 4:105-36, 1979.

Horrobin, David F., 'The importance of gamma-linolenic acid and prostaglandin E1 in human nutrition and medicine', *Journal of Holistic Medicine* 3:118-39, 1981.

Hursch, J.B., Clarkson, T.W., Cherian, M.B. *et al.*, 'Clearance of mercury (Hg-197, Hg-302) vapor inhaled by human subjects', *Archives of Environmental Health* 31:302, 1976.

Jemmott, John B., Borysenko, Joan Z. Borysenko, Myrin *et al.*, 'Academic stress, power motivation, and decrease in secretion rate of salivary secretory immunoglobulin A', *The Lancet* 1:1400-02, 25 June 1983.

Jones, V. Alun, Shorthouse, M., McLaughlan, P., Workman, E. and Hunter, J.O., 'Food intolerance: A major factor in the pathogenesis of irritable bowel syndrome', *The Lancet* 20 November 1982, pp. 1115-17.

King, David S., 'Can allergic exposure provoke psychological symptoms? A double-blind test', *Biological Psychiatry* 16:13-19, 1981.

Koos, B.J. and Longo, L.D., 'Mercury toxicity in the pregnant woman, fetus and newborn infant', *American Journal of Obstetrics and Gynecology* 126:390, 1970.

Lonsdale, Derrick and Shamberger, Raymond D., 'Red cell transketolase as an indicator of nutritional deficiency', *The American Journal of Clinical Nutrition* 33:205-11, February, 1980.

Mandell, Marshall and Conte, Anthony A., 'The role of allergy in arthritis, rheumatism and polysymptomatic cerebral, visceral and somatic disorders: A double-blind study', *Journal of the International Academy of Preventive Medicine* July, 1982, pp. 5-16.

Marshall, Robert, Stroud, Robert M., Kroker, George F. *et al.*, 'Food challenge effects on fasted rheumatoid arthritis patients: A multicenter study', *Clinical Ecology* 2:181-90, 1984.

Massod, M.F., McGuire, S.L. and Werner, W.R., 'Analysis of blood transketolase activity', *American Journal of Clinical Pathology* 55:465, 1971.

McGovern, J.J., Lazaroni, J.L., Saifer, Phyllis *et al.*, 'Clinical evaluation of the major plasma and cellular measures of immunity', *Journal of Orthomolecular Psychiatry* 12:60-71, 1983.

Meador, Clifton K., 'The art and science of nondisease', *The New England Journal of Medicine* 272:92-95, 14 January 1965.

Miller, Joseph B., 'A double-blind study of food extract injection therapy: a preliminary report', *Annals of Allergy* 38:185-91, 1977.

Monro, Jean, Carini, Claudio and Brostoff, Jonathan, 'Migraine is a food-allergic disease', *The Lancet* 29 September 1984, p. 719-21.

Nelson, Harry, 'Food allergy actually rare, science finds', *Los Angeles Times* 30 July 1980.

O'Shea, James A. and Porter, Seymour F., 'Double-blind study of children with hyperkinetic syndrome treated with multi-antigen extract sublingually', *Journal of Learning Disabilities* 14:189-237, 1981.

Pleva, Jaro, 'Mercury poisoning from dental amalgam', *Journal of Orthomolecular Psychiatry* 12:189-93, 1983.

Randolph, Theron G., *Human Ecology and Susceptibility to the Chemical Environment*, Springfield, Illinois, Charles C. Thomas, 1962.

Rapp, Doris J., 'Food allergy treatment for hyperkinesis', *Journal of Learning Disabilities* 12:608-16, 1979.

Raue, H., 'Health problems related to amalgam tooth fillings', *Medical Practice* 32(72):189-93, 1983.

Rea, William J., Bell, Iris R., Suits, Charles W. and Smiley, Ralph E., 'Food and chemical susceptibility after environmental chemical overexposure: Case histories', *Annals of Allergy* 41:101-10, 1978.

Rea, William J., Podell, Richard N., Williams, Mary L. *et al.*, 'Elimination of oral food challenge reaction by injection of food extracts', *Archives of Otolaryngology* 110:248-52, 1984.

Rudin, Donald, 'The major psychoses and neuroses as omega-3 essential fatty acid deficiency syndrome: Substrate pellagra,' *Biological Psychiatry* 16:837-50, 1981.

Rudin, Donald, 'The dominant disease of modernized societies as omega-3 essential fatty acid deficiency syndrome: Substrate beriberi', *Medical Hypotheses* 8:17-47, 1982.

Rudin, Donald, 'The three pellagras', *Journal of Orthomolecular Psychiatry* 12:91-110, 1983.

Ruskin, Asa P., 'Sphenopalatine (nasal) ganglion: Its role in pain, spasm and the rage reaction and possible relationship to acupuncture', *Acupuncture and Electro-Therapeutic Research* 4:91-103, 1979.

Sharp, Jennifer, 'Our "pipe dream" became a nightmare', *Prevention* September, 1982.

Sterner, R.T. and Price, W.R., 'Restricted riboflavin: Within subject behavioral effects in humans', *American Journal of Clinical Nutrition* 26:150-60, 1973.

Stock, Alfred, *Zeitschrift fur Angewandte Chemie* volume 39, 1926 trans. Hanson, Mats in *Journal of Orthomolecular Psychiatry* 12:202-7, 1983.

Stock, Alfred, 'Die chronische quecksilber und amalgamavergiftung', *Zahnarztl. Rundschau* 48:403, 1939.

Svare, C.W., Peterson, L.C., Reinhard, J.W. *et al.*, 'The effect of dental amalgams on mercury levels in expired air', *Journal of Dental Research* 60:1668, 1981.

Trachtenberg, I.M., 'Chronic effects of mercury on organisms', Washington, DC, National Institute of Health, US Department of Health, Education and Welfare, 1974.

Truss, C. Orion, *The Missing Diagnosis*, Birmingham, Alabama, C. Orion Truss, 1982 (available from C. Orion Truss, P.O. Box 26508, Birmingham, Alabama 35205).

Truss, C. Orion, 'Metabolic abnormalities in patients with chronic candidiasis: The acetaldehyde hypothesis', *Journal of Orthomolecular Psychiatry* 13:66-93, 1984.

Verebey, Karl, Volavka, Jan and Clouet, Doris, 'Endorphins in psychiatry', *Archives of General Psychiatry* 35:877-88, 1978.

Zioudrou, Christine, Streaty, Richard A. and Klee, Werner A., 'Opioid peptides derived from food proteins', *The Journal of Biologial Chemistry* 254:2446-9, 1979.

Zitrin, C.M., Klein, D. and Woerner, M.G., 'Treatment of agoraphobia with group exposure in vivo and imipramine', *Archives of General Psychiatry* 37:63-72, 1980.

CHAPTER 11

Hinz, Christine A., 'Winds changing for medical schools', *American Medical News* 16 November 1984

Jancin, Bruce, 'Innovative program incorporates psychiatric principles into clinical medicine clerkships', *Clinical Psychiatry News* December, 1981.

Jenkins, M.T. Pepper, 'Stop educating future doctors to be Philistines', *Medical World News* 1 September 1982, p. 124.

Mazer, Eileen, 'Prevention – Today it's "the way to go", *Prevention* December, 1981, pp. 108-12.

Nelson, Harry, 'Insurer restricts payment for new heart treatment',

Los Angeles Times 31 March 1982.

Schwartz, Harry, 'Revolt against Flexner', *Private Practice* December, 1982.

Shemo, John P.D., Ballenger, James C., Yazel, J. Joe and Spradlin, Wilford W., 'A conjoint psychiatry – internal medicine program: Development of a teaching and clinical model', *American Journal of Psychiatry* 139:1437-42, 1982.

Index